Get
<u>REAL!</u>
A Safety Guide for Women and Teen Girls

RHONDA PAYNE

ISBN:0988891301
ISBN-13:978-0988891302

DEDICATION

For the women and future women of the world. Be strong, be
assertive, be safe. For my daughter, Nikki.

CONTENTS

Acknowledgments i

1 Introduction 1

2 It's All About Prevention Pg 8

3 What Does a Bad Guy Look Like? Pg 13

4 Where Are the Bad Guys? Pg 22

5 What Does a Victim Look Like? Pg 37

6 Black Belt Body Language Pg 41

7 Trust Your Gut Pg 50

8 Physical Response Pg 60

9 Escapes Pg 86

10 Become a Black Belt in Awareness Pg 100

ACKNOWLEDGMENTS

I would like to thank all those who have shared their stories with me and those who have trusted me to teach them how to be safer through self- empowerment, awareness and training. A special thanks to Jan Bonner, who co-founded the Get REAL program with me. Her knowledge, skills, insights and passion make her the coach and instructor I aspire to be.

1 INTRODUCTION

Looking back, my life seemed to belong to someone else. That naïve kid who was so easily manipulated couldn't possibly be me. That weak, non-confrontational pleaser who let anyone with a pulse win an argument or have their way is someone else- not me. Yet, it was.

 The bright eyed optimist with the awareness skills of a rock- wanting to follow her calling in life of helping others, but being a flashing beacon of vulnerability for anyone wanting to take advantage- that's where I began. It's hard to admit that, but it's true. It seems so far away now.

 And it could be your story, just as easily as it could be millions of other women and girls stories out there. But, as the saying goes, "When you know better, you do better."

After surviving ten years of an abusive marriage, the aftermath, the rebirth of myself and over 30 years in the martial arts, I have learned a lot of valuable lessons. Lessons I'd like to share with you, the reader.

 If I can help you avoid or overcome some unpleasant or downright dangerous situations, then putting my own private stories out there will be worth the discomfort of exposing my own mistakes.
However, I am also an instructor. As a 7th degree black belt, it is my job to teach safety every day. Teaching 6-8 classes a day, 6 days a week has been my work for the past 34 years. They say we teach what we most

need to learn. I needed to learn how to defend myself- not physically so much as mentally and emotionally.

As a fighter, I could take care of myself in the ring. I had the trophies and titles to prove it. I had no fear of taking on an opponent physically. Deep down, every woman has the fighting instincts. Even the most mild mannered can turn into a barracuda if they or their loved ones are threatened with bodily harm.

Learning to develop some skills to go along with those natural protective instincts are vital to surviving an attack and walking away. However, as important as those physical defense skills are, they aren't enough. They aren't even the most important aspect of self-defense.

That's why I wanted to write this book. To teach you beyond the physical skills and address the skills you can use every single day- the emotional and mental tactics to lessen your vulnerabilities to the outside world.

Using strong body language and better communication skills, being authentic and honest with yourself about who you are, what drives you, what makes you happy and what does not-- those are the tools of self-defense! Once you no longer look, act, walk and talk like a victim, you are less likely to become one.

The sooner you learn how to project the energy that you want to put out into the world, the sooner you realize that that very energy is the exact same type of energy that you will get back. Tenfold!

Have you ever met someone who just radiates negativity? It has nothing to do with how they dress, what they look like or how good or bad they smell. It's the energy they emit. You can feel it. Literally. Negative people can leave you feeling exhausted even after just a short encounter. But, if you are not in tune with your instincts, you can stumble your way through life wondering why you keep attracting the constant barrage of negative people and bad relationships, bad luck, accidents and misfortune along the way.

The good news is it can change. You can change. Everyone does the best they can with what they have. Not having the tools doesn't make you a bad person, just uninformed. I'm here to teach you how to be stronger, more aware, more confident and safer-- physically, mentally and emotionally.

It's an exciting journey, this life we have been given. What's even more amazing is that what you focus on is what you manifest.

If you focus on the negative, that's exactly what you will manifest in your life. Not a good return on your investment. But, if you change your attitude and learn to focus on what you want, you will automatically set in motion the positive momentum that will attract positive people, situations and opportunities into your life.

It may seem strange to pick up a book about self-defense and read about energy. But, we are the result of the decisions we make whether those decisions are conscious or not. We decide **who** we are going to be and **how** we are going to be every day. Not deciding is also a decision and plays a part in our lives *and* our safety.

Throughout this book, I hope to educate you as well as inspire you- to teach you how to protect yourself, inside and out. Self-defense goes beyond physical protection. If a physical confrontation does happen in your life-- and I hope it never will or never will again-- it is but a very short event. Protecting yourself emotionally and mentally is an ongoing, everyday occurrence.

To tell you who I am now, I have to tell you some things about who I was, or, more specifically, was not. I know no one who is exactly the same person today as they were ten or even five years ago. Everyone changes, whether for better or worse, but we all change.

I began training in martial arts at the age of 15. I'd always been active in sports, although it seemed to me that I had to work twice as hard as everyone else to get even half the results. But I never gave up. I was the shortest player on the basketball team, the only hurdler who had to 4-step instead of the traditional 3-step, but I always showed up.

I gave it my best, knowing one day it would pay off. I didn't know exactly how, but I knew it was important that I try my best, even if I wasn't *the* best.

When I got into martial arts, specifically, Taekwondo, I knew I had found my calling. I couldn't get it out of my head. Everything in my life became about the martial arts. It made sense to me, both mentally and physically. I just got it. I had no idea it would become my life's work. I started out as an idealist teenager who was mature (so I thought) for my age. I was always looking for a challenge. Careful what you ask for.

I met the man who would become my husband through a martial arts center in which I was training. He was older- much, and married at the time. I was young and naïve. I thought his "special attention" was because I was an enthusiast and gifted athlete.

Looking back, I was such an easy target, mostly because I didn't know I was so vulnerable. I had a love of the martial arts, had finally found something I was actually good at, and I was being recognized for it. He was soon separated and divorced and we were married just a few months after I graduated high school. The courtship was fast and I was suddenly in the deep end of the pool with no life jacket.

Things changed virtually overnight. I went from being showered with gifts and compliments to being pelted with insults and responsibilities I hadn't signed on for. But, having gotten myself into this mess, it was my job to fix it, so I went about transforming myself into whatever I thought he wanted.

I spent the next ten years trying to be something I wasn't and not being good enough no matter what I did. It was emotionally abusive, spiritually crushing, sexually abusive and humiliating.

Emotional abuse doesn't happen overnight. Eventually the hard-edged tactics can give way to subtle comments and the abused person is like the elephant in the circus- a powerful beast being controlled by a simple rope; their spirit having been broken long ago with heavy chains when they were too small to resist. Now, they don't even try. The lesson has been learned. Fighting back is futile.

Some women, and men for that matter, never make it out of abusive situations. I was lucky. My saving grace was my daughter, Nikki, who was born about a year before I finally had the courage to walk out. She gave me the strength to leave. To start over and be the strong person I had forgotten how to be. They say mothers will do more for their children than they will ever do for themselves. For me, I know that is a true statement.

That's why I started teaching safety awareness. Not just self –defense, but awareness. If my ex had tried to lay a hand on me, I knew what to do. I could fight like a pit bull. But, this fight wasn't purely physical. It overwhelmed me at the time. It was much more powerful, too. It chained me down.

I was beating myself up even when he wasn't around. I had zero self-esteem and was told I had no options. "You can't make it without me," and "You're nothing without me," were common phrases that were ingrained into my psyche.

When you hear something long enough, you begin to believe it, whether it's true or not. And, to top it off, I had no support network around me, another classic trait of abuse: isolation.

When I finally got out, August 7, 1992 (which I celebrated as my "independence day" for many years after), I had a choice. I could be bitter, or I could be better. I decided to be better. I started reading books, which, until my divorce, had not been "allowed". For the ten years I was married there was not one book or magazine in the house. Now, my house is virtually a library!

Books are stacked in every room, including the garage and the shed. I just couldn't get enough! I still can't. I started reading everything I could get my hands on about self- empowerment, self -improvement and self- healing. I spent three years in therapy, diagnosed with post-traumatic stress disorder. I always thought that was a term reserved for soldiers, returning from a war. But, I had been in a war myself... and survived.

My first goal was to make a better life for my daughter. I soon realized that in order to make her life better, I had to work on myself first. The old saying, "If mama ain't happy, ain't nobody happy," is true. I couldn't give if my own cup was empty. Filling my cup was not selfish, it was a necessity.

Getting my life in order, physically, mentally, emotionally, financially and spiritually was not an easy task, to say the least. Some things will always be a work in progress. But, progress I did. I read once that life is like climbing a mountain: you are either climbing or you are sliding; there is no standing still for long.

Since those dark days, I have gone on to win state, national and world titles in my sport. I have owned and operated a successful business and raised a happy, healthy child who is now of legal age and can stand up for herself. She is light-years ahead of me for where I was at her age. Her future is incredibly bright.

They say sometimes you don't know what you have until you've lost it. That is true, but, for me, I didn't know how much I had lost or just done without until I began attaining. I didn't know how *unhappy* I was until I got happy. Denial surrounded me and trapped me, stifling my spirit. Denial is a powerful chain. Being unaware is so very dangerous. Ignorance is not bliss. It's costly. For me, I lost my twenties, but there are many who have lost much more. Many women have lost their lives.

Statistics say the most dangerous time for a woman is when she is leaving a relationship. Her risk for harm and possibly death increases by 75%. As we go through this book, I will give testimonials, both mine and others, who have been in a particular situation and survived. I will cite statistics occasionally, to reinforce my statements and hopefully impact you, the reader, with the importance of each lesson.

My hope is that this book will give you the tools to avoid having to defend yourself physically. But, even if you have done everything "right", as the saying goes.... stuff happens. In those cases, I want to give you the physical tools to be able to survive an attack and escape with as little physical injury as possible.

Being in martial arts, I've had many people ask me if I'd ever had to "use it." My response is always the same: Yes, I use it every day.

The character lessons, the assertiveness training, the self- confidence and the awareness I gained through martial arts I use every day to defend myself, physically, mentally and emotionally.

I've taught literally thousands of students over the past thirty years how to become more focused, be self-disciplined and achieve their goals. I am honored and humbled to have the opportunity to teach you some of these lessons. Let's begin.

2 IT'S ALL ABOUT PREVENTION

AWARENESS

What exactly does it mean to be aware? In simple terms, it means to pay attention. Easier said than done. When we are born, we notice everything because it's all new. Systematically, as our brains process each new stimulus, we dismiss those things we've seen before, heard before and felt before, relinquishing them to the mundane, the ordinary. No longer does the sound of the TV alarm us, or even catch our attention, unless there's something new or unusual about it.

We spend our days as adults eliminating more stimulus than we accept. Remember driving to work and seeing a new billboard that caught your eye? Maybe you noticed again the next few times you drove to work, but, after just a few days or so, it's lost its allure and is demoted to the ordinary file, passing by without so much as an acknowledgement. There is simply too much stimulation going on around us every day to notice it all. The key is to notice what matters.

When personal safety is at issue, it pays to notice things that will keep you safe. How can you become more aware? Like exercising makes muscles stronger, practicing awareness skills makes those skills stronger, too. Let's try an awareness exercise: If you are sitting down (NOT driving), or able to take the time to focus, try this: look around the room and pick one color, say… green. Notice everything in the room that is green or has green in it. Take about 10 or 15 seconds and take it all in. Do it now, before you go on. We'll wait.

Okay, now that you've looked all around the room close your eyes and recite everything that you saw that was yellow. Aha! You were being very aware of the greenery in the room, thus eliminating everything else. By asking for something completely different, it's harder to recall something you weren't paying attention to.

Everyone filters things in their own way. We are all motivated by different values, ideals, emotions and thoughts. For instance, if you attended a party with 10 other guests, you may have a particular instance or overall feel for the event that is completely different than the other guests' perceptions.

I have an older brother that has the memory of an elephant. He can recite the lines and characters from the commercials and shows we watched growing up that I forgot about long, long ago. It's an incredible attribute that I just don't possess. We could attend a family event, like a reunion, and he would recall the event totally differently than me. We would wonder if we had attended the same event at the same time. We had, only I remembered it completely differently than he did.

Some people are more inclined to be analytical, some more emotion based. For example, let's say there is a car accident witnessed by two people. When the police arrive and gather statements from the witnesses, the **analytically**-based witness recalls approximately what speed the cars were progressing, in which direction each vehicle was headed, how long they heard the tires screech before impact and so forth. These are good witnesses for the police reports.

On the other hand, the **emotionally**-based witness might say they "can't believe that someone would just run a red light like that and hit the other vehicle and just leave without making sure the other driver was okay." Or, "Oh gosh, I hope they aren't hurt too bad." might be a statement the emotion-based witness would say.

They can't really recall how fast the cars were heading when they collided or who hit who first or how things transpired, but they are more emotionally involved in the accident and its aftermath.

If you are the more analytical type, then noticing things out of the ordinary might be right up your alley. On the other hand, if you are more emotionally oriented, then noticing the order of things, or, when they are out of the ordinary, might take some practice. But, like any other skill, becoming more aware of such things is certainly an attainable one.

Having an idea of what to do in case of an emergency not only makes good sense, it can significantly reduce your risk of injury. Remember when you were in school and there were fire drills? The siren would go off and everyone knew their "job." Maybe you were to stand and walk in an orderly single file line to a designated spot outside the building. Maybe your job was to turn off the lights and close the door, or grab the class hamster on the way out.

Either way, you knew what your job was. It kept people from panicking, even if there really was a fire, because everyone had a plan.

If there wasn't a plan, then people would be more likely to panic and rush for an exit and possibly leave someone behind, or worse, trample them on the way out. Look at what happens at soccer games overseas. The fans rush the stadium and the people in the front get crushed.

When you panic, you lose your game plan. Your heart races and suddenly you are in a different realm of reality. When you have a defensive plan, you are still in control. You might be scared, but you know what to do. Think of defensive driving.

That's the whole idea of taking a self- defense course. You think about things ahead of time, while you are in a calm state of mind. You practice different techniques- both mental and physical until they are reflexive. Then, if you ever *have* to use those skills, they are on automatic pilot, so to speak. You might very well be scared to death, but, your mind and body will know what to do. Just like the fire drill, you have a plan.

If all else fails and you get into a physical confrontation, I want you to have a basic knowledge of what works and what doesn't. Awareness is Plan A. But, like any good plan, you need a backup. Plan B- Physical defense. We'll get into that later in the book. For right now, let's start working on our awareness skills. Here's some homework.

Humans are naturally creatures of habit. We get up, shower, dress, eat and go to school or work, or follow whatever our daily routine might be.

It may deviate to some degree, but, for the most part, it's a set routine. Now, as you go about this routine, start asking yourself this: **What if**? What if someone broke into your house while you were in the shower? Would you have a plan? What if your house caught on fire during the night? Would you know it? Would you have a plan for you and/or your family to get out safely?

The simple question of "what if" can lead to many, many a variety of scenarios. While you are in your car, ask yourself: what if the car behind me bumped me at the light? What would I do? Would I get out and inspect the damage? What if the car in front of me stopped suddenly and the driver got out and started banging on my hood and screaming? Would I have a plan?

Most times, common sense tells us what to do. But, for the sake of adding tools to our awareness tool box, I'll talk about different possible scenarios throughout the chapters.

Since every situation is different, there is no ultimate "do this exactly like I say" instruction that is guaranteed. But, life holds no guarantees either. We are just increasing our chances of survival through having planned ahead.

With that said, let me add this. Whatever decision you make in the "heat of battle"- in an emergency- is the right decision at the time. Your brain, like a computer, processed the available information of the situation and came up with a solution that was most likely to keep you safe at that moment.

It's not to say that after the fact- weeks, months or even years later- you have acquired some new information or skills that would lead you to making a different decision or handle it differently had the same situation come up today. But, it didn't. At the time you did the best you could with what you had. That's the best anyone can do.

3 WHO ARE THE BAD GUYS?

They say to win any battle you must know your opponent.

KNOW YOUR ATTACKER

No one wants to identify or associate in any way with rapists, murderers and other criminals. But, in order to avoid and/or survive an attack, we must recognize what a potential attacker is looking for and what makes them tick.

Whenever I address a group of young students or children, I start by asking them what they think a "bad guy" looks like. It's amazing to hear the responses. Here's a few-
- "He's wearing black clothes"
- "He has a patch on his eye"
- "He's carrying a sword"
- "He has guns and bombs"
- "He's ugly"

Wouldn't it be simple to identify a "bad guy" if he did look like that? Police could just go arrest the hairiest, ugliest, smelliest guy who had guns and swords strapped all over his body. Even kids think of someone who would do evil things as whatever is farthest away from whatever they are.

Unfortunately, that isn't the case. It's not what someone looks like, or how they dress that makes them a good or bad person. It's what they **do** that makes them so.

Someone that would hurt children, or assault an innocent victim-- that's a "bad guy". Ted Bundy, the serial killer, was also a very handsome and charming man. He lured women into his grasp by acting like he needed help and took advantage of others' good natures.

A major component in risk reduction is being less naïve. It takes practice, but it can be done. There is a distinct difference between being cautious and being paranoid. Paranoia is no way to live. Constant fear of one's surroundings, both environmentally and socially is not only draining physically and emotionally, it is a waste of time and energy.

There is another major factor for an attacker who is looking for a victim. An attacker is seeking someone who won't say **no**. And, as the law of averages go, if one person says no, eventually, if he keeps asking, someone is going to say yes. Or, at least, not *say* no.

One of the first things I learned studying self- defense was that rape was not an act of sex at all, but an act of violence. It's all about control. A rapist doesn't necessarily care who they harm- not their age, race or even gender in many cases.

For women, most incidences of rape and/or attempted rape are **not** stranger-oriented. Most are by someone the victim knows-- acquaintances, spouses, family members or friends. According to RAINN- (Rape, Abuse, and Incest National Network):

- 1 in 6 women and 1 in 33 men will be sexually assaulted in their lifetimes.

- College-age women are 4 times more likely to be sexually assaulted.

- 60% of sexual assaults are **not** reported to police.

- 73% of rape victims knew their assailant.

- Only 6% of rapists ever spend a day in jail.

Here is another sobering statistic. Sixty percent of rapes of girls under the age of 12 were by their own *fathers*.

On the other hand, statistically, most of the attacks on men *are* by strangers. Remember, most of the attacks on women are by someone they know.

So, the traditional "stranger danger" approach to self-defense is not, in my opinion, what is most needed. This book will certainly address those types of attacks, but it will also touch upon the subjects of domestic violence, date rape, verbal abuse, sexual abuse and more.

Rapists, burglars, carjackers- criminals in general- are opportunists. They may not have thought through the fact that they are capable and willing to commit a crime. But, if an "opportunity" arises that seems too good to pass up, they will strike. An opportunity can be anything from a car left unlocked to a woman who looks like an easy target.

By easy target, I mean someone who is either distracted or unaware, doesn't look like she'll put up a fight- or much of one- or is in a vulnerable position either environmentally, emotionally, physically, or any combination of the above.
In the case of domestic violence, the victim is   acutely aware of her attacker.

Denial is a large factor here. When the relationship started, it most likely didn't have the characteristics of abuse it took on down the road. It probably started out with a showering of compliments, attention and maybe even gifts. In the book, The Gift of Fear, by Gavin DeBecker, the author explains how attackers are quick to make a "bond" or connection with their potential victims right away.

It's like a grooming process, where they set them up to feel obligated in some way, since the attacker initially gave something, whether it was attention or gifts, and the victim feels some type of connection and obligation to reciprocate with their own attention or loyalty.

It is the taking advantage of someone's good nature that abusers thrive on. Whether they admit it or not (or whether they are aware of it or not) that's what it is. They are looking for a return on their investment.

Their investment being time, attention and/or gifts; the return being your loyalty and undivided attention or more.

When relationships turn violent, it is usually because the woman didn't follow the rules- be they unspoken or verbalized. These "rules" may have become increasingly impossible to decipher and adhere to. "You know what makes me mad" is a common phrase in an abusive relationship, as if you or anyone else has control of another human beings emotions and actions.

In my own situation, there were so many unspoken rules and regulations of what would make my spouse lose his temper that I could have carried around an encyclopedia of "rules" and it wouldn't have mattered. The rules changed according to his mood anyway. There was no way to keep up.

Realistically, it was not my fault if he got mad. I was not responsible for his emotional outbursts. But, at the time, I felt I had to change whatever I was doing, saying or being to appease his temper. I walked around on egg shells all the time, just waiting for the next explosion or argument that I would have to deal with. I thought less and less about how I felt about anything, and more and more about what I could do or not do to avoid "setting him off."

My time and energy was gradually so consumed with concerns for "keeping the peace" that I lost who I was completely in the process. It no longer mattered what or how I felt, even to me.
Recognizing abuse is one thing. Doing something about is another. I chose to stay and try and "fix it" for ten long years.

If you or someone you know is in an abusive relationship, I would encourage you to seek counsel. Get help. Quoting Oprah, "Love does not hurt." Get help getting out if that is what your instincts tell you to do. My instincts told me as soon as I got into my relationship with my ex that it was a colossal mistake. I chose to ignore my inner voice and paid the price. It was a costly lesson for me, but I did learn just how important listening to my gut was and today that inner voice is back and stronger than ever. I know of no one who regrets listening to their "gut" or inner voice, but I've met many who regret NOT listening to their gut.

I remember one conversation with my ex about how much each partner should contribute to the relationship. It quickly turned into a conversation about who should have more "say-so" or *control* in the marriage.

My answer was 50/50. He laughed. The look on his face was as if I was completely clueless- and stupid. As I WAS dumfounded by his response to my answer, I asked- what's YOUR idea- 60/40? Nope. More like 70/30. He was completely serious! His idea of what a marriage was or should be was a 70/30 split. He expected to have 70-80% say-so on any given matter. I was supposedly only worthy of 20-30% authority in the marriage. He was clear- his way and his way only.

There were so many arguments, especially early on, that were so emotionally exhausting. That exasperation led to giving in, which lead to more control on his part and less and less on mine. It was an emotional tug-of-war that he thrived on and I loathed. I just wanted peace. I've always been the peacemaker, the facilitator. I facilitated away all of my dignity, worth and value in the name of peace.

Domestic abuse is very cyclic. I experienced emotional and sexual abuse, but physical abuse runs along the same lines. There is an escalation period, where the abuser is pushing the envelope of control. It can be something trivial, like not being at a certain place at a certain time, or not having a particular task done by a certain time, or your phone rings and it's someone unexpected...the possibilities are endless.

The upward spiral begins- "Who was that? What did they want? Why? How long have you been talking to him/her? What else have you talked about? What did you say about me?" The list can go on and on. No matter how innocent the situation, no matter how truthful and harmless your response, it escalates. It escalates into a heated argument--that you lose.

All you've learned at the conclusion of all this drama and crisis is how exhausted you are. After the explosion, after the volcano has erupted and all the residual damage has been done; their seething, pouting, brewing, ignoring, fuming, stomping, etc. has settled and you've mentally and/or physically retreated inside yourself to your only safe, dark space, does the dust settle.

Only once you have given in and given him what he wanted- control- are you rewarded. You might be rewarded with a reprieve from the war. You might be rewarded with material things. It can vary. It can be a combination of rewards. But, rest assured, the volcano will rumble again. It will erupt again and it can and likely will be a more violent eruption the next time.

I remember another time when my ex's youngest son, Jason, was only 5. He was the cutest little ray of sunshine. He was spontaneous and mischievous like 5 year old boys can be. And, like all kids, he pushed boundaries. Children push boundaries to see where they are. Once they know the perimeter of their little world, they generally feel safer.

This particular instance, Jason was leaning back at the kitchen table in the metal framed chair. One of those "modern" type chairs from the 80's that were seemingly one piece of molded tubing that came down each side of the backrest and curved towards the front and back around, so there were no back "legs". He was leaning back, with his little hands on the glass top rectangular table.

He was sitting at the head of the table, dangling his little feet under the glass and being totally pleased with himself as he looked at his feet under the glass. His father, Andrew, was sitting to his right, at the long end of the rectangle. Andrew had told him several times to put the chair down. Each time, Jason complied. He'd then start to fidget again, and not long after would slip back into the fascination of seeing his legs right beneath the surface of the table.

This went on for several minutes until a fraction of an inch was passed- the balance tipped. The metal chair's corner edge met with the hard floor beyond the bottom padding and WHOOSH! Back he fell. As the chair slipped back and he was headed towards the floor, Andrew's quick reflexes kicked in. It was like watching a strange duality. In one instance, the parental instincts of a father caught Jason before he fell.

But, almost just as quickly as this father had rescued his son from danger, his anger flared. As soon as he had sat him upright in his chair, he flashed anger and struck Jason with his open hand right in the middle of his chest. His hands were "heavy" as they say. He was, after all, a high ranking Black belt and a broad-chested man. His handprint was transferred to Jason's tiny chest in a bright red, glowing split second.

He was angry for not being obeyed. He was instantly reactive and left the mark to prove it. Jason was devastated, emotionally crushed. You could see the innocence fade from his eyes. It was a milestone moment in this young boy's life. I think it changed how he looked at life after that. After it was over, it didn't really matter what type of consoling was applied as bandage. The damage was done.

I knew Andrew had remorse after the fact. But, instead of addressing it with any emotional significance, he reverted to what he knew- to buy forgiveness- to buy redemption. What was the asking price for an abuser to feel like he had "made it right" with his son? What would it take for his 5 year old son to forgive him? The 5 year old who idolized his bigger than life father? Andrew decided it would take a 5 pound bag of M&M's.

There were no apologies, no conversation about how he, as a father, had messed up or how it would never happen again. His 5 year old son was left to figure out this complex situation for himself. He was left with a 5 pound bag of candy instead of explanations. Andrew was satisfied that he had bought his way out of trouble once again. I don't think Andrew ever realized that his tactics didn't work in the long run. After 6 failed marriages, he still hadn't figured it out.

His sons all paid heavily for his temper. The emotional damage stays around long after any physical damage has disappeared. The emotional scarring from verbal abuse can last a lifetime. They can alter the path of one's journey in life. Sometimes it alters victims so severely they can't find their way back to their path at all. Sometimes they fall off the cliff.

I was 18 when I married Andrew. He was 38. His five sons from wife #1 were living with us shortly after we wed, under the veil of how we were "rescuing" them from HER.

Little did I know she was destitute- a stay-at-home mom, whose husband cheated on her throughout their marriage, who eventually left her for a younger woman: *me*. He gave her no child support. I had no idea. I'd just gotten myself into the biggest cesspool of lies and deceit imaginable. I had no idea what I was in for.

I'd been raised to be hard-working, reliable and, above all else, ethical. My shame was suffocating. I'd gotten myself into this mess; it was up to me to fix it. Walking away was not an option, at least not in my mind. I'd burned my bridges with my own parents by going against their wishes. I saw them as trying to stifle me and control me. It was a perverted, distorted view, thanks to Andrew. My mind had been poisoned. I felt alone. I was isolated physically, emotionally and he knew it.

He acted as though I was needed. I was a caretaker by nature, so being needed is right up my alley. Suddenly, there are five scraggly, hungry, hollow-eyed boys whom he's telling me NEED me. This was a challenge of epic proportions, especially since I'm only six years older than his oldest son, Andrew Jr.

Looking back, I can't believe I got so deeply involved in the drama, crisis after crisis and didn't just walk away. But, in my mind at least, I had nowhere to go. I was too young to be on my own. I had no financial independence. I had no experience. No life skills. I'd fallen into the trap of "I'll take care of you" promises that I'd been fed. I was so easily bought it was pathetic. A few shiny things and I was mesmerized. Lures. Baited- Caught- Trapped. Easy prey.

Within a year of being married, I was stepmother to five. Cooking, cleaning and caring for children whom I had no authority to parent, no decision- making rights. Yet the physical responsibilities for taking care of these boys fell on my shoulders most of the time.

I'm not telling you my story to air dirty laundry or get it off my chest. It's been many years since I was the malleable, young idealistic girl with the disease to please. I am telling you these stories in the hope that you can identify in some way with the circumstances.

If you are being used, manipulated, abused or taken advantage of, I want you to learn from my past. I overcame all the trauma, drama and abuse and got out. It took ten long years. Ten years of trying to "fix it".

Ten years of negotiating, bending and finally breaking to realize that I could only be responsible for myself. I blamed Andrew for a long, long time. All the things he did and the things he did to me.

But, ultimately, it was my choices that got me where I was. Just like the choices I make today shape me for tomorrow. It was up to me. It was up to me to get out. It was up to me to make sure my daughter was not raised in that toxic environment. It was up to me to be responsible for myself. My decisions, my happiness, and my safety- it was all up to me.

I know for a fact that I wouldn't be who I am today if I'd stayed any longer. By the time I left, I had gotten to the edge of the cliff and the choices were clear: Kill him- kill myself- or leave. **So** glad I took door #3.

4 WHERE ARE THE BAD GUYS?

KNOW YOUR ENVIRONMENT

Making and keeping yourself safe to avoid attacks is priority one. An ounce of prevention is truly worth a pound of cure. Some things on each list may be something you already do; some things you might not have considered before reading this book. Either way, take from it whatever you need and begin to implement them into your life. Nothing happens overnight when learning new skills, so don't try and do everything all at once.

Home Checklist:

- Make sure and lock all outgoing doors each time you come and go. I know this sounds simple enough, but, burglars have repeatedly stated that they chose the houses they burglarized by which one was unlocked.

- If your front door doesn't have a peephole, have one installed.

- Never feel obligated to open the door, even for someone you know. Most friends, family and guests do not show up unannounced. You might have to train them to call ahead, but,

22

it's for your safety-- and theirs. Anyone who cares about you will not be offended that you asked them to.

- If you don't already have deadbolts on exterior doors, get them. Replace shorter screws in the strike plates with longer ones, like 2.5 or 3 inch screws, the kind that will go into the framing and not be ripped out as easily. If you have chain locks, make sure those screws are replaced with longer ones, too.

- When closing the blinds, think of where someone might try to see through. Turn the horizontal type blinds concave side out if you are at a higher elevation, say 2nd story window and higher. For ground floor windows, turn convex side out so anyone across the way who is higher up can't see down in.

- If you don't have an answering machine, get one. Screening your calls is not rude. Anyone with good intent will leave a message and be glad when you call them back at your convenience. Many people don't even have a home phone; they just use their cell phone as their main number. These all have caller ID. If you don't recognize the number, you don't have to answer it. They can leave a message.

- If you have someone who is stalking you or calling repeatedly, use a digital message, instead of your voice for the recording. Your voice might be just what they want to hear. A digital recording is more impersonal, but that's the idea. Again, those with good intent won't be offended in the least.

- Keep all windows locked. It might be the coolest breeze tonight, but it's just not worth the risk.

- If you have a sliding glass door, like a patio door, keep a stick or dowel that is just a bit shorter than the opening and lay it in the track. This will prevent the door from being opened. Make sure it is no more than about ¼ inch shorter than the opening. You can always attach something to it to get it out more easily. A quick solution is to staple a string near the end so it's easy to lift up.

- Make sure your windows and exterior doors are not cluttered visually by large shrubs or bushes. Don't make it easy for someone to hide.

- For ground floor windows, many people prefer to plant thorny shrubs and cactus underneath the window to make entering especially difficult.

- Make sure you have a deadbolt on the door leading from your home into the garage and keep it locked at all times.

- If you park your car in the garage, consider these options. When leaving, get in, lock your doors and then lift the door. When arriving home, pull in, shut the door after making sure no one followed you in and then get out. It may take just a few extra seconds to complete this scenario, but it is time well spent. Keep your doors locked until the garage door is completely down. Many garage door openers have a safety mechanism that will automatically stop the door from closing should someone or something cross the threshold before it is down. In those cases, the door will automatically go back up.

- If you find yourself in a situation where someone has entered your garage, back out and start honking your horn. Use your cell phone to call 911 and do not exit your car. Drive to the nearest safe place, whether it is a local police station, gas station or store that is well populated.

- Have a security alarm and motion detectors installed. At the very least, get some window stickers and a yard sign. Burglars who are looking for an easy target may just pass you by.

- If you live alone, you don't have to look like you do. Light timers can make lights go on when you aren't home. Dogs are great for barking when someone comes around, too. If you don't have a dog, get the biggest dog dish you can find and lay a well chewed, super-sized dog chew near it. Maybe your neighbor has a dog that could do the honors.

- If you are going on vacation, be sure to stop the paper delivery. Nothing says "I'm not home" like a stack of newspapers in the driveway.

- Do NOT plaster on Facebook that you are leaving on vacation! Social media is great to keep in touch with family and friends, but it's not the place to tell everyone that you won't be home.

- Get to know your neighbors. Having someone look out for you and you for them is invaluable. Have their phone # saved in your cell phone registry.

Work

- Workplace violence can happen at any company. Listen to your instincts!

- Leave your building in pairs or groups whenever possible. Many larger companies have security guards on duty that will walk you to your car.

- If you must close at night, lock all doors while you are inside alone. If your company keeps cash and/or controlled substances on site, be sure to have escape plans in place should someone break in.

- If you go on calls, such as a real estate agent or home health care, be sure to let others know who you will be meeting, where and what time. Get their information ahead of time and leave it at the office. If you arrive first, note the car, license number, etc. before you exit your vehicle.

- Lock your purse and valuables in a locking file cabinet or locker during the day. Whether it's the general public or other employees, keep your things less vulnerable.

- If someone crosses your personal boundaries, whether through inappropriate talk or behavior, report it to the HR (Human Resources) person in your building. It can be done on a confidential basis. If there is no such department in your company, at least take it to a higher authority so they know what's going on and it's documented.

- If someone doesn't take no for an answer, an immediate red flag should go off in your head. Distance yourself from them as soon as possible.

SCHOOL

Children are by nature, very trusting individuals who look for the good in others. It's a good quality to have, but it is also a vulnerability that predators take advantage of.

One of the first things to teach children is how to say no to an adult. It contradicts most of what they have been taught all their lives. But, knowing *when* it's okay to say no is crucial.

Most things in a child's world are black and white; there is no gray area. When we explain things to kids, they sometimes interpret very differently than we think. Even with the best intent, things can get blurred.

For instance, I teach martial arts to kids. Many years back, I was preaching how, in martial arts, we learn how to fight so we don't *have* to. Bullying would not be tolerated, nor would fighting at school. The intent was to teach kids that walking away from a fight took more guts than fighting. However, when I had a young student come to me and tell me how he had been beaten up at school, I had to reconsider my approach to teaching certain values.
Now, this was not a small kid. He was big for his age and he was an advanced belt, so I knew he could handle himself.

As the story went, he was being picked on by a smaller boy, but thinking that he would be kicked out of class if he was caught fighting, he took the abuse, even when it became physical. He loved participating in martial arts so much that he would rather get beat up than not be able to participate in class! I felt horrible! I felt like the worst teacher on the planet. We had a long discussion about how defending oneself is not the same as getting in fights. If someone is attempting to hit you, by all means, defend yourself.

I learned a big lesson that day-- at the expense of my student being punched-- that I had to explain things more thoroughly and make up for the lack of gray area in kids interpretations.

When I teach self- defense to kids, I try to explain it in a way that they can understand. If an adult approaches them and asks them to do something or help them in some way, then a standard response should be this: "Let me ask." The standard rule is: an adult never needs your help. They shouldn't be asking you to help them find their missing pet, fix something, or give directions. The child should go immediately to the nearest adult or safe area. Make space between them and the adult as quickly as possible.

Here's a story that happened several years back. There was a young girl, about 11, who was playing in the apartment complex where she lived. A man approached her and said that he was having trouble with the washing machine in the Laundromat and asked if she could help him.

Being a normal, compassionate kid, she followed the man. He then abducted her, duct taped her mouth and put her in the trunk of his car and took her to a remote cabin in the woods and assaulted her for the next two weeks. By some miracle, he brought her back and dropped her off near her home. He was later caught trying to abduct another young girl and was shot and killed by police. In his vehicle, they found a fake badge, a dog leash, handcuffs, duct tape and various items he had used to lure young children into his grasp.

He was responsible for a rash of abductions throughout Texas and several other states. He had picked up kids at their bus stop, on their way home from school and, in this case, an apartment complex.

The young girl who was abducted and held by this maniac had been very resourceful over the extent of her ordeal. Even though she had been traumatized by this man, she made a point to remember the various sounds she heard while in the trunk of the abductor's car and the approximate length of time she was in the trunk which helped lead the police to his hideout. She also saved some of his beard hairs he had cut off while in the cabin in his attempt to change his identity.

She had his DNA in her pocket when she was rescued and she assisted the police in narrowing the field of where his hideout could be. She was lucky to be alive. Some of the other victims that this man abducted were not so lucky. Police found the body of a young female victim on the cabin property.

Encourage children to speak up. Setting and keeping healthy boundaries takes practice. If an adult asks for help, kids should not feel obligated to help them *themselves*. The "let me ask" policy gives kids permission to get away and go to the nearest trusted adult.

There is nothing more sacred than being trusted with health and well-being of a child. To cross the boundaries of this trust and rob them of their innocence is not only a sin, it is a crime. I don't care what field you are in-- whether you are a teacher, a coach, a priest, a counselor or any other capacity-- taking advantage of children is deplorable and unacceptable.

Just today, as I was preparing to write, a well-known Catholic priest made the news as his comments about pedophilia in the church were aired and then later removed and replaced with apologies. This guy was not only a VERY well-known priest and TV show host, but also holds a Ph.D. in psychology from Columbia University!

To think that an institution as large as an entire religion has been covering up cases of misconduct and pedophilia for so many years is despicable. Part of his comments referred to the Sandusky scandal, where the Penn State Coach who was later convicted of child rape was referred to by this priest as "poor guy," making the argument that teachers, priests, etc. should not be sent to prison on their first offense. Incredible!

They may have taken this guy off the air and published an apology, but he's not the first to try and cover up either his own past or the past of others who have manipulated children and taken advantage of the position they held.

A typical justification from a child molester, or from a rapist, is that the victim somehow "wanted it" or provoked it or it was somehow the victim's fault that this happened. That is such a lie! It is NEVER the child's fault! The shame on the part of the victim, the cover up on the part of the offender and the lack of transparency on the part of whatever institution or agency that is in charge is the reason it perpetuates.

Yes, children should speak out. It can stop the abuse and punish the offender. But, it is incredibly difficult for a victim to take a stand who has been taken advantage of, made to feel like it was somehow their fault, told that they won't be believed if they do tell, humiliated, and hurt, even when they are adult victims. Children should be protected. Period.

It is not their responsibility to protect themselves from pedophiles-- it is society's. It is not their responsibility to see that justice is carried out-- it is society's. The only way to stop the abuse of children is for the tolerance of it to stop and those who commit these types of crimes are punished-- *severely*.

- Adults never need the help of a child. Not for directions, not for help carrying things, not for help looking for a lost pet. These are all tactics used to take advantage of children and "good strangers" won't ask.

- The standard answer kids should learn when asked by an adult other than their parents, is "let me ask." This gives them an out and lets the adult know they are not going to go easily.

- Practice speaking up drills with your kids. Role play "what if" games and coach them how to handle various situations. Being assertive takes practice. And praise from parents.

- Be on the lookout for signs of change. When an outgoing child suddenly becomes quiet, when eating habits or sleep patterns change, when friends and social circles change or stop altogether, or when one person seems to dominate their time and attention. There's a reason for everything, but sometimes we need to look a little deeper and not dismiss changes as "just a phase", unless it truly is.

- Bullying is an enormous problem in the school system today. But, it goes beyond school grounds. Bullies grow up and get jobs and continue to harass and demean those around them. Teach your children to speak up. To tell you, the parent when things are happening that make them feel bad. To tell the teacher and keep telling until something is done. To tell the bully to stop. All of the awareness skills we need as adults, we need as children, too. Positive self-image, confidence, assertiveness-- those are tools of self- protection.

THE COLLEGE YEARS

College-age females, ages 18 to 23, are the largest group of rape victims. For these women, it's not stranger related rapes that top the list. It's date rape. For young women who are typically away from home for the first time in their lives, living more independently than they ever have, making their own rules as to when and where they go and whom they go with, it's that first burst of freedom that can get them in trouble.

There are so many new experiences for college kids. Socializing is a big part of college life. It's a chance for young people to spread their wings and discover who they are. Unfortunately, it is also a time for drinking and partying beyond reason for many. Date rape happens both on and off campus. And, for many young women who have been victims of rape and assault, they are ashamed to report it to the authorities.

Even when they do, many are re-victimized by the very organizations that are there to protect them.
There is still a stigma attached to women when it comes to date rape or sexual assaults. To ask a woman what she was wearing, as if that was an instigator of the attack is insulting. To ask her if she wanted it, or if she'd done it before is degrading. It doesn't matter. It doesn't matter if she was drinking, or if she was intimate with the perpetrator before. No means no. Period.

Whether the victim knows the assaulter or not, whether she's dating him or married to him, it doesn't matter. No means no. No matter how many times she's said yes before. No means no.

It's a woman's perfect right to wear whatever she wants to wear, go wherever she wants to go and talk to whomever she wants to talk to without fear of being raped. But, in the real world, women have to be aware of where they go, whom they associate with and what they wear.

It's unfortunate that women have to watch their drinks when they go to a club for fear that someone will put something in it. It's unfortunate that women have to let someone know where they are going and who they are going with just in case they don't make it back.

It's unfortunate that women don't feel safe to walk across campus or across the street without looking out for who's looking at them. But, they do. They have to. It's a part of life to be aware. Aware of your surroundings. Aware of the little voice inside that tells you to pay attention. Aware of the subtle changes that signal the evening, the date, or the encounter is taking a turn for the worse. Aware of when it's time to move away from someone who is making you uncomfortable before it escalates into something more dangerous. Aware of when it's time to be more assertive.

Aware of when you need to speak up and speak out. Aware of when you need to involve more people in order to get the help you need.
There are lots of things women need to be aware of. It's learning to be aware and not paranoid that makes life go more smoothly.

Getting in the habit of letting your roommates know where you are and what time you will return isn't too hard to master. Getting in the habit of confiding in someone you trust gets easier the more you do it.

Getting in the habit of expecting men to treat you with respect and not tolerating anything less is not only going to make you feel safer, but it's going to make you feel more confident, which is going to make you safer.

If you are the victim of date rape, whether it's on a college campus or not, it is your right to go to the police and report it. It's not your fault.
Get some support for yourself and report it. Don't worry about whether anyone will believe you or not. Keep talking until you get the help you need. Every college campus is different, but they should have some kind of campus police to help deal with assaults and criminal behavior. If not, call the police and get help. Keep talking until you get the help you need.

It's your right and you deserve it. And, by speaking up, you could very likely be helping prevent future victims. If someone is willing to sexually assault one woman, they are capable of hurting more- sometimes MANY more. The sooner they are stopped, the better.

The statistic is that fewer than 6% of rapists spend a day in jail. This is mostly because it goes unreported. Regardless of whether or not a rapist is convicted or sentenced, the act of standing up for yourself and reporting it can help start the healing process for the victim.

By acknowledging what happened, reporting what happened and not allowing it to happen again, the victim is more able to get past it and move on. When we deny things and try and stuff it down inside by not talking about it, not processing it and not allowing the healing to take place, it's like swallowing poison and expecting the other person to die. Talk, get it out. Get the help you need if you are the victim of a crime. Once you do that, you are no longer a victim: you are a survivor. You are able to move forward and leave the darkness behind.

SHOPPING

Whether it is seasonal shopping or everyday shopping, there are plenty of opportunities for thieves to take advantage of the crowds. Next time you go to the mall, look around and see if you can spot the easy targets.

You know who they are. The woman in the food court at the mall who hung her purse over the back of her chair and never thought how easy that made it for the passing thief to help himself. The lady that didn't bother to zip or close her purse, but threw it over her shoulder. The shopper that didn't bother to put the laptop in the trunk, but left it in the back seat, along with the tablet, or the golf clubs, or the shopping bags, or……

While you are out spending your hard-earned money, you shouldn't have to worry about others trying to take it, but a little awareness can go a long way to staying safe and making it back home with everything you left with as well as all of the cool new stuff you scored on your trip.

While you are making your way back to your vehicle with armloads of goodies, think about your vulnerabilities through the eyes of the bad guy. Are you looking around as you walk, or are you unaware of your surroundings? Are your arms so full you couldn't react to someone trying to grab you or your things, or do you look ready, with one free hand to deal with any challenges?

Did you park close to the store in a well-populated area, or are you trying to get your exercise in and hoofing it all the way to the end of the lot? What does a bad guy see when he sees you?

TRAVELING

The world may seem a little smaller these days thanks to the internet, but it's still a long trip to get from LA to NY. Whether you travel by plane, train or automobile, good awareness and a little prevention will make your trips more enjoyable as well as safer.

Having your itinerary mapped out can make your trip go smoother, but having your eyes open to what others see when they see you is paramount to staying safe.

Having a bad plan is still better than having no plan. With airport safety, everyone knows that you have to get to the airport in plenty of time to wait in line, have your belongings inspected, take off your shoes, go through the metal detector, etc. Be prepared to wait, be prepared to carry whatever you decided to drag along with you further than you anticipated.

Be prepared to spend time with people you'll likely never see again. Be prepared if someone becomes cranky or irate or even violent in your presence. It happens. It doesn't happen often, but it does happen. Well, the cranky part may happen quite often, but the violent part not so much.

Ask yourself, "What if?" What would you do if someone treated you disrespectfully? How would you react if someone became physically violent? What would you do if someone tried to grab your purse and run?

Knowing ahead of time what you are willing and capable of doing in any situation lessens the anxiety in the event it does happen.

I'm not talking just about physical violence here. I'm talking about any encounter. Write down any situation you can think of that would make you feel uncomfortable, anxious, defensive or unsafe in any way.

Then, role-play with yourself or even with your trusted friend what you might do in any given situation. Maybe try out 2 or 3 different responses and possible outcomes in order to broaden your perspective. The more prepared you can be mentally, physically and emotionally, the more positive the outcome you can produce.

I remember years ago hearing some speaker talk about dealing with road rage. I can't remember who it was, or I'd give him credit for it, but it went something like this. When you are driving down the road and some jerk cuts you off and flips you the bird, don't lose your cool. Just think, in fifteen minutes you'll be where you were going, having forgotten all about it and the other driver will still be a jerk!

You don't have to take on someone else's negative energy. Recognizing that their bad behavior is a reflection on them and not on you can help you to not take it personally.   It's not about you, it's about them; therefore it's their problem- not yours.

Your job when you are traveling, or any time for that matter, is to keep yourself safe. Be aware of what is going on around you. Listen to your gut when it tells you to pay attention.

SOCIALIZING

In this age of internet connections, there are more and more relationships that start out online. There are chat rooms, groups and all kinds of ways people connect. If you meet someone online and decide to take it to the next level- a face to face meeting- be diligent about your safety.

The dating protocol of today is very different than in years past. If you are going to be meeting someone, especially for the first time, there are a few rules to consider. First, meet them somewhere neutral. A place where you are comfortable either way. If the date goes well, you've been somewhere you enjoyed. If the date goes sour, then you are surrounded with potential help, witnesses and outlets for escape.

Second, get there on your own accord and leave on your own accord, when you want to. If you have someone pick you up, you relinquish control as to when and how you leave.

Third, let someone know what's going on. Let someone know who you will be meeting, where and what time you expect to be home. This information can be more valuable than you realize if something bad does happen.

Not to say that something bad will happen, but if it does, being just a little prepared on the front end can save a lot of grief on the back end.

Besides, if who you are meeting is potentially someone whom you would date, then why be elusive about it with your best friend? Not only can they share in your safety, but they can share in your joy if it turns out well.

5 WHAT DOES A VICTIM LOOK LIKE?

VICTIM PROFILE

Victim: *(According to Webster)*
one that is acted on and usu. adversely affected by a force or agent <the schools are victims of the social system>: as a (1) : one that is injured, destroyed, or sacrificed under any of various conditions <a victim of cancer> <a victim of the auto crash> <a murder victim> (2) : one that is subjected to oppression, hardship, or mistreatment <a frequent victim of political attacks> b : one that is tricked or duped <a con man's victim>

Simply put, a victim is someone who is taken advantage of. It can be as simple as being in the wrong place at the wrong time.

The other definition of a victim is someone who won't say no. Attackers and abusers alike look for victims who don't say no.

Remember, they are looking for the best return on their investment. If you don't put up a fight, or much of one, then you are a prime target. If you don't set and keep personal boundaries, then others will gladly walk right past them and take advantage of you.
Avoidance is the best game plan, so being aware of your surroundings, what potential attackers are looking for and what you are doing are key factors to staying safe.

THINK AHEAD

Whenever possible, plan ahead. They say failing to plan is planning to fail. Some people just seem to be born with planning and organizing skills. Unfortunately I missed that line when they were passing those genes out. Even though it is something I have to consciously practice to improve on, planning ahead and organizing *is* possible and you can improve, too.

Those "Type A" personalities that we've all met seem to have it down to a fine science. They go on vacation with full itineraries of "fun." I can't say I have an internal "to do" list that is quite as long, but it is there. Since I am more of an "in the moment" kind of soul, I tend to be in the present most of the time. It is a conscious effort for me to think longer term, but, when it comes to personal safety, it is a must.

Review the checklists from earlier. If you see something(s) that you could improve upon, then start with one thing and gradually increase until you've checked them all off of your list. Any new habit takes time to implement-but consistency is the key to success. Not perfection, but consistency.

WINDOWS OF OPPORTUNITY

Burglars, rapists and criminals in general are opportunists. Remember back when cars didn't have alarms or those "clubs" for the steering wheels? Most cars were stolen by being broken into to back then. When the car alarm came along, it slowed the traditional break-in and car-jackings skyrocketed. It was easier to get into a car with someone already *in* it, than to get past an alarm, or a club.

Think of it this way. There are two cars parked side by side. One car is a Corvette, shiny and expensive, but it has an alarm and the doors are locked. Car #2 is a junker, with dings on the side and a paint job of primer and rust. But, car #2 is unlocked and the keys are in the ignition. Which car do you think the opportunist will go for? The nicer one that is going to involve more time and risk to attain, or the easy target? Chances are, it's car #2 that's going to get stolen.

The same goes for leaving things of value in plain sight. If there is a bag in the back seat or something that looks like it might have value, a car thief will not hesitate to bash in your window and help themselves to your stuff.

One of my students told me about his parents' truck being vandalized because there was a brown bag on the floorboard. It turns out that it was just a bottle of wine, but the thief couldn't tell what it was before they broke the window and took it. It just looked like it could be of value.

If you can stash it in the trunk, do so. If not, try and hide it completely under the seat, out of sight.

Our training center was for many years located in a shopping center that had a liquor store next door. Ironic- there was a bar, a liquor store, our training center and a day care all in the same center. It went from being full of children during the day to being full of drunks at night.

There were several occasions where we witnessed a liquor store patron go in for "just a second" and leave their car running-- unattended. The same thing happened frequently at the convenience store at the end of the shopping center. On more than one occasion, cars were stolen. The opportunity was just too much to resist.

Leaving a car running, unattended is just asking for it to be stolen. There was even a car stolen while a dad was inside the store and his young daughter was left in the car. Thankfully, the daughter was retrieved safely, but it could very well have ended tragically.

The key here is not to make it easy for someone to steal your stuff! Make yourself and your belongings a hassle to steal, abduct or abuse. Those looking for an easy target will move on to the next one. Better to be called a name or given a dirty look than to be a victim of crime.

6 BLACK BELT BODY LANGUAGE

Your body language is the unspoken conversation your body has with the rest of the world, without you saying a word. As a fighter, reading my opponent's body language was critical. I could tell what they were going to do before they did it. If they made a certain movement, I knew what they were going to throw and I had a counter attack ready. It was an integral part of a winning strategy.

You read others body language all the time, whether it's a conscious thought or not. If you walk into a room and see your child with a certain expression or demeanor, you instantly sense their mood. If someone in line at the grocery store gives you a certain look, you instantly feel a certain way.

Most of the time we dismiss it because it's not sending up a red flag of alert. We all make assumptions and judge others every day; we just dismiss it so quickly it doesn't make an impact. When you see someone or meet someone, countless thoughts flash through your brain instantly. Tall, short, cute, ugly, nice, gross, clean, dirty-- the list goes on and on. We don't typically think too much about it happening, since it's been going on all our lives.

A potential attacker uses the body language of those around them to weed out those who look like they would be too much trouble and hone in on those that look like the easiest targets. Let's take a look at some aspects of body language.

POSTURE

Posture says how you feel without you saying a word. When you feel good, your body reflects that. Your back is straighter, your head is held higher and you look stronger. When you feel poorly, your posture reflects that, too. Confidence shows-- and so does a lack of confidence. Lack of confidence is just what an attacker or potential abuser is looking for.

Along those same lines, let's talk about personal appearance. It is your perfect right to wear whatever you feel appropriate. But, the reality is, the more provocative the clothing, the more attention it is going to draw. Whether it is tattoos, expensive clothes, eye catching bling, or cleavage, it is going to draw attention.

Be prepared. Have a plan ahead of time for how to handle wandering eyes, comments, pick-up lines and unwanted attention.
Again, practice in your head, practice in front of a mirror. Practice in front of a friend-- however you want to do it, just practice.
How would a strong, totally confident, take no B.S. kind of woman handle it? Visualize it. Feel it. Fake it till you make it. I'm not saying you have to change who you are and turn into someone else. But, when the circumstances change, you have to change.

I am the friendliest person you could happen to run into under most circumstances. But threaten my loved ones, threaten me and you will see an instant transformation from poodle to pit bull. It's like flipping a switch. Now, it doesn't have to go that far; it could be as simple as changing your facial expression to show that you mean business. It could be changing your posture, showing your awareness of the situation that can de-escalate something before it even begins. That's the best outcome-- to stop something before it starts.

EYES

The most expressive of your body language- your eyes- can say how you are feeling in an instant. Whether joy or anger, your eyes can flash your mood like a bull horn. Use it to your advantage.
If you are walking down the sidewalk, make confident eye contact with those you pass by. Avoiding eye contact or looking down gives others the signal that you are not confident. Making eye contact acknowledges that you see the person. Not glaring; just acknowledging their presence shows confidence. Look around as you walk. Pay attention to what is going on around you, as others may be paying attention to you.

Like anything else, it's easy to say and hard to do for some people. So, if confident eye contact is not in your nature- at least not yet- then practice! Stand in front of the mirror and act "as if." If you were the most confident, assertive person you'd ever met, what would that look like? Practice keeping your head up, shoulders back and walking and looking confident. Walk around the house feeling like you just won the World's Strongest Woman contest, or the Olympic Gold in Judo, or the MMA world title.

Look at yourself in the mirror as if you were the number one chef, teacher, artist, doctor, lawyer or Indian Chief in the world. What would that look like? Act as if! Emit the energy of a strong warrior. You ARE a strong warrior! Even if you haven't realized it yet.

PACE

What does your pace say when you walk? Too fast a pace tends to relay nervousness. Too slow- distraction. A confident pace is one that looks like you know what's going on around you, you know where you are going, and you know who is around you. You are present, in the moment. The last thing an attacker wants is someone who is ready for them. They lose their element of surprise if you are paying attention.

GESTURES

If you have ever been around someone who was an animated storyteller, you know what this means. They talk with their hands. They are the "touchy-feely" type. You never want to get too close because you might get slapped, pushed or poked. Again, use this to your advantage.

The distance that you can extend your arms is your close range comfort zone. No one should get within your range without your permission. If someone attempts to get too close, use your body as a "fence" to keep them out. Get your arms out in front of you in a defensive posture and turn slightly sideways. Steel your eyes, straighten your back and look like you'll put up a fight. Words such as "Back off!" or a simple "NO!" can deter an attack.

There is a book called Beauty Bites Beast, by Ellen Snortland. It's a great book. I recommend you read it. Although it's been many years since I've read her book, the story she tells of her trip abroad still stays with me. She talked about traveling to Japan to do a safety seminar. As she was standing in the train station, she noticed a group of school girls in their uniforms also waiting for the train. Then, she witnessed an old man- apparently drunk, stumble to the group of girls, who, in their culturally polite habits, didn't defend themselves when the old man groped and touched them. Even as they giggled uncomfortably, they didn't try to stop him. He made his way through this group of young girls and stumbled up to Ellen.

As he approached, she took a defensive stance, with her hands held out in front and fingers spread apart and yelled "NO!" At that point, the startled old man, stumbling backwards-- eyes wide open in surprise-- started to make his way back to the group of young girls.

As he neared this group for the second time, one of the girls took the same defensive stance she had just witnessed Ellen successfully defend herself with and yelled something in Japanese-- probably the equivalent of NO!-- and the baffled old drunk did a double take. He stopped in his tracks, looked at the girl, looked at Ellen and then stumbled his way in the other direction. The young girl, not speaking the same verbal language as Ellen, had just learned from her body language how to defend herself-- and it worked!

TONE

The tone of your voice changes with your emotions. When you are calm and relaxed, your voice takes on a soothing pace and tone. When you are agitated, your voice reflects it. If your house was on fire, would you whisper softly to get everyone out? Of course not! You would scream at the top of your lungs with the urgency needed to get anyone and everyone's attention.

In a self- defense situation, taking your voice to a deeper, more commanding level can be quite effective. Say something like you mean it.

I remember watching horror movies as a kid and thinking how pitiful the women were. They always screamed these high-pitched, annoying screams and cowered down while the villain easily overtook them. They had a mousy, high-pitched voice that commanded no authority at all. They looked and acted helpless. They were victims, and it showed.

Homework:

Try standing in front of the mirror and looking at yourself. What is your posture? Does it reflect confidence? If not, try and stand "as if." If you were the most confident creature on the planet, how would that look?

Now, look at your eyes. Are they intense? Try squeezing your brows together and raising one brow higher than the other. Remember when you were a kid and were fascinated with your facial expressions?

Think of every emotion that you can, good or bad, and try and express them in the mirror. Does what you feel reflect in how you look? What do people see when they see you?
Now talk to yourself as if you were talking to someone else.

First, talk gently, like you are talking to a friend. Now, more assertive, as if you are the boss. Now, *forcefully,* as if you are telling someone to stop who is crossing your personal boundaries. I know this sounds a little strange, asking you to stand in front of the mirror and pretend. But, if you aren't or haven't been in touch with your own self-concept, it's a good way to practice. And, practice makes perfect, so go ahead. As you do this, you'll see things that look different than they feel. Once you notice them, you are more able to change what you want to change and reinforce what you do well already.

In the corporate world, videoing oneself to improve on speaking skills is a regular routine for many. Organizations like Toastmasters help people learn to be better speakers. It's a great tool in confidence building. If you've never done that, I'm sure there's one near you or something similar that you can get involved in and start improving your presentation skills.

MOTION CREATES EMOTION

When your body is in motion, the blood flow is better, therefore more oxygen is getting to and from your brain. More oxygen means clearer thinking. Most people think better on their feet, while moving around than while sitting.

Moving is also a great way to create space. If someone is invading your comfort zone, get out of there. Give them the space.

The closer someone is, the more opportunity they have to lay a hand on you and potentially control you. The more space between you, the less control they have.

If you are sitting, and someone makes you uncomfortable, don't hesitate to get up and move. If you move and they continue to follow you, then a more defensive posture and tone may be required.

By moving, you are either going to be away from the potential danger, or, at least, more aware of it.

DEVELOPING "BLACK BELT BODY LANGUAGE"

In martial arts, black belt is the Eagle Scout of ranks. It is a highly respected and honored rank, signifying years of dedicated hard work and self-discipline. When I ask my students what a black belt is, they yell back in unison "a white belt that never gave up!" Everyone starts as a beginner. What makes a black belt, or anyone successful at any endeavor, is the tenacity to never give up. That tenacity breeds confidence. Not arrogance-- there is a difference. Arrogance eventually will bite you in the proverbial behind. Confidence won't.

As I teach a martial arts class, many times I ask my students "If you were a black belt right now, how would you be sitting?" Immediately, the response goes from being slouched to board-straight backs with eyes widened. Essentially, it is a mind-set. I tell them, if you want to *be* a black belt, you need to *act* like one, *think* like one and *train* like one.

That mind-set is what helps manifest success.
The same goes for personal protection. It's not about changing who you *are;* it's about changing your mindset. You have to know, in your heart, in your gut, that if something happened and you had to defend yourself or loved ones that not only would you be *able* to do it, that you **would** do it. It's a survivor mentality.
Just like those who survive cancer, tornadoes, hurricanes and accidents, survivors all possess the same thing--a survival mentality. They made up their minds that they *needed* to survive and they *will* survive, no matter what the odds.

There was an elderly woman in Florida whose car was hit by a drunk driver late at night as she was driving on a bridge. When she was hit, her car swerved and went over the bridge, landing upside down and hanging in a tree over the swamp below. For three days, the woman hung there, upside down, with broken bones- as snakes and mosquitos crawled about. A cleaning crew was making an unanticipated early sweep through the area when a worker noticed a car had gone over the bridge and was down below.

They rescued the 80+ year old woman and amazingly, she survived the ordeal with little effects other than dehydration, a broken arm and bug bites.

After interviewing her later, she retold her tale of taking her niece to the airport for a late night flight and was coming home when she was hit by a car on the bridge.
She knew if she died, that her niece would blame herself for the accident, so she *had* to survive. She had a survival mentality.

Make up your mind today, right now, that if something horrible happened to you, that you have reason to survive. No matter what the odds, you **can** survive-- you **WILL** survive.

There was a news story years ago about a woman who survived cancer. Now, I know that if it's my time to go, it's my time. There's nothing I can do about it. But, if it's not, I'm going to do everything I can to survive and thrive.

This particular woman was diagnosed with some extremely rare form of nasal cancer. The doctor told her that only 1% of the patients who were diagnosed with this form of cancer survived. Her response was immediate. She said, "Well, then, I guess I'm that 1%!" And survive she did.

The interview was years after her diagnosis and it had been in remission for some time. That is survival mentality in action!

7 TRUST YOUR GUT

Intuition: (Webster's definition)
1   :   quick   and   ready   insight
2 a : immediate apprehension or cognition b : knowledge or conviction gained by intuition c : the power or faculty of attaining to direct knowledge or cognition without evident rational thought and inference — in·tu·i·tion·al \- ˈish-nəl, - ˈi-shə-nᵊl\ adjective

How many times have you listened to your gut and been wrong? Chances are, the times you've been wrong is when you *didn't* listen. We all have senses. The ability to see, hear, taste, touch and smell are our five senses we rely on every day. Intuition is our 6th sense.

 Everyone has the ability to sense danger before it happens, or sense when something is about to change or occur. Some are more sensitive than others; some are just more in tune with their own intuition, but we all have it.

Like a muscle that gains strength through exercise, our intuitive skills increase and become stronger when we learn to listen and trust ourselves.
Have you ever been thinking about someone and they call soon after? Have you ever gotten a feeling about someone you just met? Have you ever had the thought cross your mind that someone was looking at you

and, upon looking up, someone was. That's intuition at work. It's going on all the time; we just don't always pay attention to it.

If our inner voice tells us something, it seems to start out as a whisper. If we don't pay attention, it can go away, but, when it comes to our safety, it usually raises its voice. The whisper can become a shout, with hair standing up on the back of our necks and chills running down our spine. Our whole being is in "fight or flight" mode.

Again, it's there to protect us. It is cuing us to pay attention. What information we gather after the fact is how we decide on our next course of action.

I remember one time going out to dinner with my daughter and a friend. It was a typical Friday night as we entered the Chinese restaurant, just like almost every Friday night. It was our weekly treat to our favorite eating place.

We knew the hostess and were familiar with the family-type atmosphere. But, this particular time it just seemed a little different. A little off, although we couldn't put our finger on it. We had even discussed it at the table.

As with any restaurant, we typically choose a table or booth that is near some kind of exit, but our backs are to the wall and we have a clear view of the front door. This particular restaurant had a checkout counter by the front door and the staff had their personal belongings behind the counter. Around the corner in the dining area, was a large group of people who seemed to be family, eating together.

There were some very young children at the table and some older adults as well as two young men, maybe in their early twenties. As this "family" finished their meal, the women and children exited the restaurant without fanfare. A few minutes later, there was some screaming and a father/son at a table near us jumped up and ran out of the restaurant.

When they returned, they filled us in on what had happened. Apparently, after the "family" had left, the two young men began to pay their bill. When the hostess opened the cash register, one of the young men reached over and helped himself to the cash in the drawer while the other reached around and grabbed whatever purses he could grab and they both ran from the restaurant into a waiting car.

The "family" car! Even though there were small children and grandma aboard, the adults were all in on the deal.
The father/son duo at the table near the front heard the commotion and witnessed the event and went running after the thieves. They didn't catch them, but did get a description of their vehicle and recorded their license plate number and gave a statement to police.

Afterward, we talked about how different the air seemed when we went in. Nothing was going on and nothing had happened, yet we could feel it was different. It confirmed for us just how powerful our intuition can be.

"CREEPY PHIL"

You may have heard about a California man, Phillip Garrido who, along with his wife Nancy Garrido, abducted an 11-year old girl, Jaycee Lee Dugard as she was waiting at her bus stop. Garrido held little Jaycee captive in his backyard as his sex slave for an incredible 18 years and fathered two children with her. He was a convicted sex offender, wearing an ankle monitor and held this girl for almost two decades in his own back yard!

The car that was used to abduct Jaycee was still on the property and neighbors, who called Garrido "creepy Phil" had alerted police to the fact that they had seen children in his back yard.

This pervert was apprehended by two college campus police women whose intuition was heightened by Garrido's peculiar behavior. He had come to UC Berkley requesting space rental for a religious revival. Apparently, he was starting his own religion and carried around a box with which he professed to speak to God.

Accompanying him were two young girls. Suspicious campus police then ran Garrido's profile and found that he was a convicted sexual offender who was prohibited from having any contact with children. He was arrested and confessed to fathering the two young girls with Jaycee.

What is incredible about this story is that he was a monitored sexual predator **and** neighbors had reported him. It took the heroism of two officers to listen to their gut and pursue it further. They didn't just dismiss it-- thank goodness. Garrido is now being investigated for two other abductions and the possible serial killings of prostitutes.
A dangerous man is off the streets thanks to the two courageous women who listened to their gut.

"What you are thinking you are becoming." -Henry Ford

We know already that what we focus on, whether negative or positive, is what we bring into our reality. You are basically going to find whatever you are looking for. So, if you are looking for the worst in someone, chances are, you are going to find it. The same is true for the opposite.

The attitude of gratitude is so powerful. It's amazing, and it works. People self-sabotage all the time. For whatever reason, they don't think they are worthy enough, they don't think they deserve to be happy, they don't think they deserve to be treated with respect and dignity. Whatever the underlying cause, it will consciously or unconsciously sabotage their happiness and safety.

They do this by looking for the worst in someone who treats them well. They distrust someone who is good to them and gravitate towards those who abuse them. That abuse can be subtle or blatant. It can be the "friend" that gossips and creates crisis and drama. It can be the relative who dominates others by intimidation or aggression.

For me, there were several friends and family members who tried to intervene on my behalf early on, before and after my wedding vows. I was so closed off to them that their words and concerns never got through to me. Not that I didn't feel it; I knew they were right. I knew I was in a bad space and unhappy and scared and feeling trapped. But, in my mind at least, the thought of mustering the energy it would take to turn this situation around was overwhelming and too much to fathom.

I didn't know how to explain it. I felt like it would take God Almighty himself to be standing there with me to make this bad situation change. The feeble humans standing before me were no match for the Herculean hold my abuser had on me. In reality, it was me that didn't have the strength to fight back.

For me, outside validation was a key factor in my ability to stand up for myself and say the words "I want a divorce." I sat with my sister-in-law and talked about how unhappy I was and how I didn't want to live that way anymore. I don't remember the words of the conversation, but I do remember another human being telling me it was okay to feel the way I felt, and that it was okay to change.

It seems strange to me now to think that I couldn't make a decision on my own, for my own benefit as well as my daughter's, without some outside validation. It doesn't matter. It was what I needed to finally get that last push and topple that boulder over the cliff, that boulder that had been smothering me all those years.

Whatever it takes to get in a positive state, in a positive environment and making positive forward motion is worth it. For me, it was a relief to hear someone else tell me that I wasn't crazy, that I wasn't alone and that I was right to feel the way I felt. It gave me strength.

I knew I had to be the one to take this challenge on and do all the things it was going to require to be free of this marriage and this man for good. I knew it was going to be a hard row to hoe, so to speak, but I was filled with renewed hope and energy-just by being validated. Now, I was already out of the house and staying with my parents. But, I had done that before. According to FBI statistics, a woman leaves an average of seven times before she leaves an abusive relationship for good. SEVEN times!! I had left before. I had left before my daughter was born, I had left, but I always went back.

My mental state was weak and he had a hold on me that wasn't broken by distance. He'd call and say something that he knew I wanted to hear. "I'm sorry." "I'll change." I think I just didn't want to be a quitter. Back then, I was still in the frame of mind that I had to "fix" it. Whatever "it" was. My marriage. Him. But, it wasn't up to me to "fix" him.

By quitting, or leaving, I felt like I was being defeated. But, my spirit had been defeated and crushed for years already. By getting out and divorcing this man who disrespected me and abused me, I wasn't quitting at all. I won! I got my life back. And I won a life for my daughter that she would NEVER have had if we'd stayed.

They say the definition of insanity is doing the same thing over and over and expecting different results. I finally got it. My "AHA" moment. I couldn't change him. I could only change me. So I did. And it was worth it. It was *so* totally worth it.

I have experienced such an incredibly good life that I wouldn't have if I'd stayed stuck in the past.

I still, after over twenty years of being gone and done with that whole mess, am giddy sometimes when I do something fun and wild and crazy and spontaneous. I can get up in the middle of the night and go out into my studio and throw pots on my wheel if I want to. I can go anywhere, do anything, talk to anyone, wear anything I choose and not worry or check my back.

There's no one to tell me I'm not allowed to do this or that. I can eat what I want, when I want, with whom I want. I don't have to "answer" to anyone but myself. That is my right. And it is your right, too. Back then, I gave up those rights. I had to fight to get them back, but it was my biggest win.

HOPING VS. EXPECTING

Just like having a survivor's mentality is critical to overcoming obstacles in life, the difference between hoping and expecting can mean life or death in a self- defense situation.

Hoping means you have no control over the outcome of a given situation. Expecting means you play a part in the outcome. This is where men and women seem to differ immensely. For instance, let's say you are standing by the curb at the airport, waiting for your ride.

You have just finished an exhausting day of travel and meetings and can't wait to get home. The sun is just beginning to set and it is getting dark rapidly. From across the parking lot you spot a less than savory man walking right in your path.

What goes through your mind? "Oh God, I hope he doesn't come over here." If that is your response, then you are *hoping* he doesn't come over and ask you for money or want to talk to you or whatever. You have no control over the outcome.

On the other hand, if it were a man standing there waiting for a ride, do you think that "Oh God" thought goes through his mind? Do you think his heart races the same way a woman's does with the anticipation of danger? I think not. Even if the guy is only 4 feet tall and weighs 100 pounds soaking wet, he is more likely to pump up his chest, make solid eye contact with the approaching male and give off the testosterone stare.

You know the one: the look that says "You don't want any of this, buddy". That guy is expecting the outcome of the situation to end in his favor. He is playing an active part in his own safety.

Call it machismo, call it whatever you want. It works. It's a mindset. Just by looking tough, it is often enough to send an approaching troublemaker on to the next potential victim instead of wasting their time on someone who might put up a good fight. As the old saying goes, "It's not the size of the dog in the fight, it's the size of the fight in the dog that matters."

Go from poodle to pit bull in an instant if you have to.

ANXIETY VS. DANGER

We all have anxieties about one thing or another. Some are inherent, some are learned. It's good for us to have some healthy fears. Fear of fire, fear of moving vehicles and the like. It keeps us healthy and alive.

What we fear in those instances is danger. Something real- getting burned, getting run over- those are very real dangers.

Anxiety, on the other hand, is the feeling of fear when there is no imminent danger present. For example, I had a friend who had driven safely for many years with no accidents or incidences to speak of. On one particular car ride, she and her husband were involved in a horrible accident where a car coming from the opposite direction crashed into the car in front of them. As their own vehicle began to roll, they saw the boat that was being trailered behind the car come sailing over their heads and land on the car behind them.

They both walked away from the incident with minor injuries, mostly from the air bags and seat belts, but my friend was so traumatized after the ordeal that she had nightmares and extreme anxiety for months afterward about riding in a car. There was no imminent danger, but her anxiety prevented her from going about her daily routines.

Let's take a scenario and look at the difference between anxiety and danger. You and some friends are at a club and you have a strange feeling that something is not right. You have just left an abusive relationship and aren't used to being out on your own with no one to answer to.

You keep looking over your shoulder, almost expecting your ex to come barging through the door and demand you leave with him. You can't relax and have a good time because of your pre-occupation with the notion that your ex will know where you are and show up. That is anxiety.

Now, if you are at this club, and your ex, whom you have a restraining order against shows up, then, there is a real danger present. That is not anxiety; that is danger.

For me, the first scenario was real. I had just filed for divorce and my brother, his wife and some friends decided that I had some catching up to do. They took me out to "have a good time" and I was miserable. Not only was I anxious about my ex showing up; I hadn't done the club *scene.* I got married just months after I became "legal".
I found out two things: first, I don't enjoy clubs. It's just not my thing. Second, I was feeling anxiety, not danger. I didn't have a restraining order against my ex and he didn't have a clue where I was and I knew that.

But, I was out of my comfort zone and my mind raced with possible threats.
It was several months before I could go anywhere comfortably without looking over my shoulder.

The anxiety and residual effects of a bad relationship can be crippling. It takes conscious efforts of rational thinking to get out of constant "survival mode" into a relaxed state.

Living in a state of crisis is exhausting. When you are in danger, your body and mind react to that danger by going into the "fight or flight" mode. It is designed by nature to heighten your senses for a short period of time. The caveman had to decide whether to run from the dinosaur or stay and fight. In a self- defense situation; you must decide the same. But, to live in a constant state of anxiety is not only exhausting, it is useless.

If you are constantly afraid to walk from your apartment building to your car or the bus stop, ask yourself this: how many times have you walked that route? How many times have you walked that route and been attacked?

If you have unfortunately been attacked, was it once or every day? If you have lived in your apartment for 2 years and worked 5 days a week, that's roughly 260 days of work, so that means you left and returned to your apartment some 520 times just with work related excursions. How many of those times did something bad happen? Odds are, not many, if at all. So, the key is to pay attention, not be paranoid when you come and go.

8 PHYSICAL RESPONSE

SECONDS COUNT!

The first seconds are the most crucial.

The initial contact is when an attacker has the least amount of control. Therefore, the first seconds are the most crucial. The longer someone has contact with you, the more control they can gain.

Whenever an attack occurs, it is best to finish that confrontation right where it began. When it comes to crime, a secondary location is almost always a deadly one. Wherever an initial attack occurs, you can bet it is better than being dragged off to a more remote and isolated location where a victim has even less chance for escape and/or help.

If you are attacked, do NOT let yourself be taken to a secondary location. It literally can be a matter of life or death. Fight, scream, do whatever you have to do to get away, but do not go to a secondary location.

If you are in your car and someone pulls a gun and demands you drive them somewhere, get out if you can. Take off without them; scoot over to the passenger side and get out, or drive your car into an object like a building or another car. Do not get taken to a secondary location.

If you are confronted on the street, make noise and get attention. The last thing a bad guy wants is to get caught. If he tells you not to yell, then he is telling you what he doesn't want you to do, do it! Yell at the top of your lungs!

 What he doesn't want is to draw unwanted attention to himself and the situation. If he wants to rob you, then he wants to get your property and get away without getting caught. If he wants to kidnap you, he wants to do it as quickly as possible, before anyone can help you. If he wants to rape you, he doesn't want anyone to interfere.

Think of it this way. If you were going to steal a car, would you do it while there was a police officer next to it? Probably not. You would want to maximize your chances of successfully stealing that car. Anything that would slow you down, or get you caught is what you would be trying to avoid. So, if someone is assaulting you, they don't want to get caught. They want to do their business and leave. You, as the victim can slow them down with yelling, screaming, kicking, punching, poking and generally not cooperating.

If someone wanted to steal your wallet or purse, then throw it one direction and start running in the opposite direction. If they are after your merchandise, then they have no reason to pursue you.

A popular tactic for thieves is to wait and watch for people who live in apartment buildings. As they are getting their keys to open the door, someone will run up, grab the purse and run. It is a surprise attack. The element of surprise is what an attacker is counting on. They don't want to confront someone who is ready for them. Being alert and knowing what is going on around you is invaluable.

Lisa, a lady that took our seminar, gave a testimonial about being in a parking lot, in her truck, and witnessing a man assaulting a woman right in front of a store. She began to honk her horn and attempted to draw attention in order to make him stop beating this woman. The man looked up at her and immediately charged for her truck. He tried to open her door, but it was locked.

It startled her, but she kept honking her horn. Store employees eventually came out and restrained the man until police arrived. It turned out to be his wife that he was assaulting. If Lisa hadn't locked her door, she was sure the man would have assaulted her, too.

One of the most powerful weapons an attacker uses is fear. It can be crippling. Women stay in abusive relationships out of fear, either for themselves or their children, or both. Pedophiles keep their juvenile victims silent out of fear. Whether it's fear of rejection, fear of reprimand, fear of injury or death, or fear of being shamed, fear can damage the victim as much as the assault.

Rape victims often do not report their crime out of fear. This lack of speaking up and speaking out only assists the perpetrator in getting away with the crime, often, time and time again. The FBI reports that a typical child molester has an average of 112 victims. An *average*!

One victim speaking up and stopping an attacker can potentially save many others from the same horror.

If you are a parent, the last thing you want to think about is someone harming your child. However, according to FBI statistics ,the reality is that one in four girls and one in nine boys will be sexually assaulted in their lifetimes. How can this be?

Often times, sexual predators are not horrible people to be around. They can be charming, funny, and- here's the key- accessible. Many child sex offenders have access to kids. It's not necessarily a stranger who is molesting kids.

Most likely, it is someone they DO know. It is typically someone who spends a greater amount of time around children. Over the past 10-15 years child molestation in the church has come to light and is no longer taboo to talk about. The astounding number of molestation cases has shed light on a horrible crime that has gone unpunished for too long.

Molesters can be someone who you trust: family members, friends, coaches, teachers or neighbors. It is important that you listen to your instincts if you feel that your child has been molested, or is being groomed for molestation.

Basically, grooming is a process child molesters use to get their victims guards down. They may spend lots of time with the victim- giving them gifts, taking them places- all in an attempt to bond with them so they will be less likely to "tell" on them later. Fear and shame are big protectors of rapists and molesters.

If your child or another child acts suspiciously, or "cries out" to you, that is, they confess to you about an incident, the best way you can help them is to stay calm, listen and not pass judgment or get defensive.

It is incredibly hard to speak up about something as horrible as being raped or molested. Thank them for trusting you enough to tell you. If they are not your child, then you can decide how to go about telling their parents, and involving the police. It is non-negotiable that the police should be involved.

The only way to stop the cycle of violence is to speak up. If a child has the strength and courage to speak up, then the adults around them should have the courage to protect them.

My hairdresser, I'll call her Terri, gave me her testimonial when I went to get my hair done. I was telling her about our safety program and asking if we could leave some brochures in her salon.

She started telling me about how being molested as a teenager had been the root cause of her many years of anorexia, bulimia and drug use. Terri is happily married with grown children. I was shocked, yet not surprised by her story, since I have heard it told similarly by many women over the years.

At the age of 7 or 8, she remembered lying in her bed and her older cousin, who was visiting with his family, came into her room and got on top of her and starting fondling her as she pretended to be asleep. Just then another family member came down the hallway and the boy abruptly stopped and left the room. The incident was never spoken of between them, nor was the boy reprimanded in any way.

Then, when she was 13, Terri spent the night with her best friend. Her best friend's father began molesting her over the course of several months. He had apparently been molesting his own daughter as well. He wasn't violent; he was manipulative. Terri spent many years being angry, getting in trouble and dealing with drug and alcohol abuse, anorexia and bulimia.

It was at a church retreat some 25 years later that she finally broke her silence and let the healing begin. The damage caused by her rapist was far reaching, but she has made it through the darkness, thanks to her faith, her courage and her family's support.

Terri is one of thousands of women who have had to deal with the effects of being raped. Worse yet, she was just a child who was raped by an adult, whom she trusted.

Anyone who is entrusted with children, and violates that sacred trust, should be exposed and punished to the fullest extent of the law.

Children are the weakest of the herd, and it is up to the adults around them to recognize danger and help protect them against it. It is never too late to speak up. It doesn't matter if it happened 50 years ago. It is never too late to break the silence.

Although rape and sexual violence occurs mostly to women and girls, it is not exclusive. Men and boys are subject to violence, too. One of the grandparents of my students recanted to me how he avoided being kidnapped as a teenager. This man was in his 70's when he told me his story. When he was in high school, he was walking home after a basketball game at school and a truck pulled up alongside him and the man inside, whom he didn't know, said "Hey, neighbor. Would you like a ride?"

Assuming he *was* a neighbor and the fact that his house was another mile down the road, he gladly accepted and got in.

As they drove, the man passed the gravel road that was his exit. An uneasy feeling came over him as he realized his driver was heading towards the highway. Remembering what his father had taught him, he reached over and pulled the keys out of the ignition and tossed them out the window.

As the driver was struggling with steering a vehicle that was no longer running and had locked up, the boy jumped out the passenger side, rolled onto the gravel road and ran several miles home without looking back.

He didn't tell anyone what had happened or how he had come to be scraped up, from his jumping out of the truck, until about a week later when another boy showed up at school having had a similar injury and incident. He then told his parents what had happened, who contacted the police.

PRACTICE MAKES PERFECT

When you practice any skill, you will improve. Role playing is a way to practice verbal skills, just like sparring is a way to improve fighting skills. The more you practice, the more confident you become. The more competent you become and the less vulnerable you become.

Here's a game you can play all by yourself. "What if?" What if the guy in front of me in line starting making inappropriate comments to me or to the little girl behind me? Would I say something? What would I say? How would I handle it?
 Would that work? What if it didn't? What if it escalated to physical violence?

What if my husband came home and lost his temper? How would I handle it? Would I engage him or would I leave? Remember, if anyone lays their hands on you, there is a zero tolerance rule, so if you ask, "What if they hit me or grab me?" the answer should always be, "Get out!"

You have to love yourself enough to get out. You have to respect yourself enough to get out. From someone who has, as they say, "Been there, done that", I can tell you that the light of day is SO much brighter after getting out of that storm I called a marriage. No one deserves to be humiliated, degraded, abused or hurt.

It's so hard to see past where you are sometimes, but, in the case of abuse, getting out is worth the effort. I thought it would actually be harder than it was. I had bought into the line of crap that my ex was feeding me. "You can't make it without me. You can't survive on your own. You need me."

What I actually found was that I was a strong woman! I could and did start my own business and thrive. I could pick myself up and dust myself off and start over.

When I left, I took my daughter, our clothes, one dresser and the only vehicle that was paid for, an old, beat up Ford pickup truck. It had no air conditioning, no power steering and a hole in the 2nd gas tank. But, to me, it was a Mercedes!

My daughter and I bounced around in that old piece of junk like we were queens riding a bumpy throne! She'd fall asleep in her car seat, holding onto my arm, sweating in the Texas heat, but we were happy! Sundays were a big day for us. I'd save up my change and we'd go to Taco Bell for Taco Sunday! Pitiful, I know. But, it was a big deal back then. It was something special that we both looked forward to. Taco Bell was the only thing I could afford to "splurge" on.

I think what I was so excited about was the fact that I could go anywhere I wanted- ANYWHERE! Anytime. I was free. We were free. I was free to raise my child in a way that I could be proud of, in her best interest. I could make decisions and not have to worry that my authority would be overruled. I could put my foot down and it stayed! My daughter once told me that I was her mother AND her father-- that she did just fine with one parent. I cried. It was a victory for both of us that I got out of that abusive relationship.

But, I have to say, it took me a while to learn how to be good to myself. I wasn't used to listening to my own instincts, let alone trust them or act on them. It took practice. I had given up so much of myself that I didn't even know what I liked!

When I moved in with my parents, I moved back into my old room. I had a small, adjoining bathroom with a sink and a toilet. I made a pact with myself that whenever I got a few dollars, I would buy myself something special. It sounds weird, but I had not had any personal products to speak of before that.

Sure, I had the essentials: a toothbrush, toothpaste, deodorant and a brush. That was about it. Now, I could spend MY money on what I wanted. It became an adventure! I bought hair spray, mousse, gel... before I knew it my little sink counter was filled with toiletries! It was my own personal stash of special things that I'd never had.

Collectively, the total price of what was on my counter space was probably worth about $25- maybe. But, to me, it was like I'd spent my lottery winnings on myself!

Now, I don't know if you've ever been as far down as I was or not. But, it took conscious effort for me to raise my self- esteem. I started with buying some personal items for myself. Then, I started making a date with myself. Yep. Once a month, I set aside a day, or an evening that I did something nice for myself-- just because.
If I had money to spend, I might buy myself a CD- (I love music!). If I didn't have money to spend, (which was more often than not), I treated myself to a bubble bath, or a walk in the park, or something that I really felt was a big deal. It was a private journey I had to take myself through.

I started with once a month, then gradually moved to once a week. I haven't had to "set a date" with myself in many years. I have so much to be grateful for these days. But, in the beginning, I had to take baby steps. I think the reason I needed to write this book was so that I could show women, you, somebody out there, that if I can do it, so can you.

If I could survive, so can you. Honestly, this book started out as a physical self-defense book. Not that those types of books aren't important- they are, but, it wasn't MY book. My purpose. My calling. I think part of my purpose is to show others that it can be done. You CAN get out of a bad relationship. You CAN rebuild your life. And, it can be greater than you could ever have imagined!

If someone had told me in my twenties that I would be living in the house of my dreams, driving a nice vehicle, owning my own corporation (!) and doing what I love to do, having won National Championships and a World title, I would have told them they were crazy. I couldn't see it then.

But, I've done all that and more. I've raised a strong, well-adjusted child who didn't have to witness her mother being humiliated, over- powered and degraded during her most formative years. I've parented the way I wanted to.

I know now that we are exactly where we are in life as a direct result of the decisions we've made up to this point. I spent ten years in a miserable situation. Not because my husband abused me but, because I let him. I allowed it to happen. I allowed someone to disrespect me. It wasn't because he was a bad guy- he was- but that's not it. It was because I participated.

I wasn't stupid; I was taken advantage of. I needed to learn the lessons, so I got the course I attracted and chose. They say the strongest steel is forged in fire. I made it through the fire and I am stronger because of it. I wouldn't be who I am today had I not been through what I have.

I've been a very private person when it comes to my emotions. I've helped many, many people deal with theirs over the years, but I've never truly shared mine. But, as I approach my 50's, I think it's time. It's time that I share my story so that others can learn.

I was very honest with my daughter from the start. I've always told her two things: One- do not ask me anything you don't want to know, because I will always tell you the truth. There are some things we didn't discuss until she was over 21, but she always got an age appropriate, truthful answer. Two- if you can't talk about it, you shouldn't be doing it.

Communication is such an important part of our lives. It's lacking in many instances and could solve and prevent a lot of trouble and heartache for a lot of folks. I can't say that I'm a great communicator.

But, I do know the importance of those two values I taught my daughter.

I hope you'll give those two items some thought. I hope you will consider implementing them into your life. I hope you can lead, or learn to lead, an authentic life. Be yourself. Be true to yourself. You deserve the best this life has to offer. Don't be afraid to make mistakes- that's how you learn. But, learn. And keep learning. And growing. You are the most unique flower in the world. Go blossom.

THE INITIAL CONTACT

As I stated earlier, the initial contact is when the attacker has the least amount of control. The longer you engage, the more control the attacker can gain. This can be interpreted two ways. One: Physical contact. An attacker's ability to control you physically.

The longer they have you, the more dangerous it is for your safety. If an attacker can take you away from the initial scene of the crime to another, more remote location, it is almost surely a deadly location.

If you are physically attacked, then deal with it right there, not somewhere else. You will have more opportunities for escape and getting help from the scene of an initial attack than from a secondary location. Put it in your mind now- no matter what- do NOT let yourself be taken away from the scene of the crime to a second location.

Scream, fight, run- do whatever you have to do, but do NOT go to a secondary location.

Two: Verbal contact. The ability of the attacker to manipulate you through purely verbal interactions. The longer you engage with someone who makes you either uncomfortable or unsafe, the more dangerous it can become.

Many physical attacks begin with verbal manipulations. For instance, many abusive relationships started out with verbal manipulation on the part of the abuser. First, they shower their new love with compliments and gifts, slowly going from asking probing questions, such as, "where were you when I called" to demanding and expecting answers to account for your every move.

This can also be the case in a workplace environment and not a relationship. There are many times when women will put up with a creepy co-worker who doesn't respect their personal boundaries. Afraid of "rocking the boat" or losing their job, women can be the victims of office-place harassment, or violence by continuing to engage with someone whom they fear or loathe. If you are being harassed by a coworker, there is no reason to let that continue.

If you cannot separate yourself from the person or situation, then it's time to go higher up the food chain and get some help. Try the human resources department, the boss or the boss's boss-- somebody down the line of authority who can help you needs to know what's going on.

Sometimes there seems no way out of certain situations. There really is, but it may take some creative thinking and enlisting the help of outsiders to either change the environment or get you out of that environment all together.
Sometimes things are not always as they appear. In the heat of the moment, or at the time, a situation may seem insurmountable. But, there are many situations I can look back on years later and see a simple solution one way or another. But, at the time, I was in crisis, less knowledgeable or whatever- and I couldn't see the forest for the trees, so to speak.

If I'd gotten help or had fresh eyes look at the problem, the outcome may have been different. It's the same for anyone. I can recount many situations where the fatalistic approach of not being able to see past wherever I was got me in trouble. I was more afraid of the unknown than whatever I was dealing with. I knew how to cope with what was going on at the time, even though it was a mess of a situation to be in, I knew how to deal with it. The thought of a complete change into something unknown was overwhelming and crippling at the time.

Many, many victims stay because they are more afraid of the uncertain and unknown outside of their own little world than the hell they live in. Even though it can be 1000 times better if they leave, they just don't realize it.

NEVER BELIEVE ANYTHING AN ATTACKER TELLS YOU

An attacker is in it for themselves and they do not have your best interest in mind. Period. Don't believe them. Don't believe them when they say they won't hurt you if you don't scream. Don't believe them if they tell you they'll let you go if you just_____.

 Don't believe them if they tell you that it's your fault. Countless children are molested under the controlling lies of pedophiles. Lies that keep children from telling of their abuse for fear they may jeopardize their family's safety if they tell. Lies that keep victims silent for fear they will be blamed for what happened, or continues to happen.

When I speak to children about personal safety, I always let them know that it's not their fault. If someone has taken advantage of them, it's not the victims fault! It doesn't matter if they were gullible, or naïve or they cooperated or they didn't fight back. It's not their fault. It is the fault of the attacker.

 There is no deadline on speaking up about abuse. It could have happened yesterday or it could have happened many years ago. There is no reason to carry the burden and take the blame. Don't accept it any longer.

FIGHT OR FLIGHT

To Fight or Not to Fight, that is the question...

If someone wants something that you have, such as your purse, your wallet, your car, it's a material thing that can be replaced. Nothing material is worth your life.

If someone attacks you and wants your "stuff," give it to them! You can always get new stuff! You can't get a new you. I tell my students that if someone put a gun to my head and demanded the keys to my car, I'd give it to them. I have insurance! I can get a new car. It's not worth the fight. If someone wants your money, literally throw it one way and run the other direction. If it's really the money they are after, then it gives you a small window of opportunity to get away. Take it and RUN.

DO OR DIE TIME

When it comes to self- defense, the best fight is when there is no fight at all. If you can avoid a physical confrontation, that is optimal. Whether you have done everything right or not, sometimes, a physical confrontation can happen anyway.

If a situation occurs, you have to make a decision whether to stay and fight, or escape immediately. If escaping is an option, it's always your best option. However, you may not have that opportunity, at least, not right away.

Since every situation is different, there is no way to say absolutely how to handle it. But, know this- whatever decision you make is the right one. At the time of an incident, your brain will (or has) processed all of the available information and come up with the safest solution for you at the time. Your brain is in survival mode. It wants you to survive.

Many times, women will second- guess themselves after the fact and feel guilty about the decision that they made in the heat of battle. Know this, the decision you made at the time was the best you could do with the information you had. Feeling guilty, feeling like you made a mistake in how you handled things will do no good. You did the best you could at the time.

Learning new skills, whether physical, mental or emotional will enhance your skills for future events, but will not change the past.

Having said that, let's get back to thinking ahead. Always be looking for an escape route. If the building you are in suddenly caught fire, have you thought about how you would get out safely? If you are driving your car, have you thought about how to avoid an accident if another car enters your lane?

As a driver, you don't consciously go through possible scenarios every moment you are behind the wheel. But, if something occurs, you have a basic game plan. It's called defensive driving. Think of self -defense the same way. When you first learn something, like driving, you may be nervous because you lack experience. Especially when you are learning something new, it is hard to relax when you are trying hard.

Unfortunately, there is no shortcut for experience. But, as you do gain experience, you gradually relax and things become more efficient and proficient. Think of any sport or craft you have learned over the years. As you gain experience, you begin to develop your own style and flow. Things that you may have struggled with initially seem effortless when you have more experience.

Learning to be aware of your surroundings, reading people, recognizing potential danger- these are all skills that develop through conscious thought and effort. Eventually, these skills become second nature and you will do them with seemingly little or no effort.
Women are endowed with a wealth of gifts and talents that we may take for granted.

Never underestimate how powerful we are as women. Use the gifts that you already have and enhance them to your benefit. If you are a gifted speaker, use that talent to de-escalate a tense situation. If you can't run or get away, then improvise. Negotiate.

Scramble until you can get free. If it is merchandise an attacker wants, then give it to them. Whether it is your purse, your wallet, your keys or your clothes- let it go. You can always get new "stuff". You just can't get a new you. Throw it one way and go the other way.

According to the Department of Justice data, the chances of getting shot at by a gun wielding attacker are small. Only 2% of victims who run from a gunman get shot. Of the 2% that got shot, only 2% of those had fatal injuries.

So, if someone is unfortunate enough to have a gun drawn on them, the chances of getting away are 98% for those who run.

WEAPONS

The more intelligent you are, the longer you'll hesitate to use a gun. Would you use it?
The choice of whether or not to carry a gun must be a well-thought out, personal decision. If you are not willing to use it, then don't get one.

Most states have handgun laws. In my state of Texas, there is a concealed carry law whereas you must be licensed to carry a concealed handgun. A safety course and a background check is part of the process.
Statistically, it takes an attacker about one second to cover some 9 feet. So, if someone kicks in your door, you have very little time to get to your gun, take it off of safety, aim and fire.

If you are going to carry a gun, I strongly recommend that you get some training. Go out to the range and practice, practice, practice.

If carrying a gun is one of your options, then be a competent, responsible and confident gun owner and user.

Several years back, there was a teacher, Diane Tilly, who was killed with her own gun. She had hired a man, Ronnie Joe Neal, who had solicited his lawn care services door to door to do some yard work at her home. He had a teenage daughter, Pearl Cruz, with him when he worked and Ms. Tilly had given them lemonade and made small talk with them, even offering a child's swing-set to Neal.

Several days later, her doorbell rang. She answered the door and it was the teenage girl, Pearl. She asked to use the phone, as she was having car trouble and Diane Tilly welcomed her into her home. Once inside, Pearl pulled a gun on Ms. Tilly, forcing her to the floor, and let Ronnie Joe Neal, her father, a convicted burglar and robber, inside her home. The two ransacked Ms. Tilly's home. They stole jewelry, found Ms. Tilly's handgun and took her ATM card. She gave her attackers an incorrect ATM pin number as she tried to stall.

As Pearl held a gun on Ms. Tilly, Neal actually left and came back. After the first failed ATM attempt he threatened to kill her dog and fired her gun into her couch. She then gave him the correct pin and he left again. Upon his return, he put a pillow case over her head and repeatedly assaulted and raped her.

After several hours, the two attackers forced Diane Tilly onto the floorboard of her Cadillac and took her to a muddy field and shot her six times, leaving her to die. Pearl later told police that as Ms. Tilly cried out in pain and begged for her life, she prayed for Pearl, saying, "Bless this child." Her body found some two weeks later, wearing only a tee shirt from the school where she was a well-respected and beloved teacher.

Pearl Cruz struck a deal with prosecutors and led police to Ms. Tilly's body, which had lay in a muddy field covered with brush.

Ronnie Neal's 15 year old daughter had been an accomplice in this horrific ordeal. As it came out later in court, he had been raping his own daughter for years and selling her for sex on a regular basis. She later gave birth to his child. She had been a victim for years and was so brainwashed by this man that she assisted in Diane Tilly's death. A tragedy in more ways than one.

Ronnie Neal had planned his attack on Ms. Tilly. She was a target because he thought she was rich, and she was nice. He took advantage of her good nature. Ronnie Neal later died in prison while awaiting execution.

YOUR BEST WEAPON- YOUR VOICE

In my training center, I teach the children that their best weapon is their voice. If you can't be bigger and you can't be stronger, then you have to be smarter.

Self-defense is about using what you have. Use what you already possess, use what is around you, or make do with what you have. Your voice is your alarm. There are many sounds that you can produce.

A mother instinctively knows when the sound her child makes is one of anger, or pain, or fear. The difference in the tone is apparent to her. In a public situation, the sounds one makes cannot be as easily determined by strangers. Making an "emergency" sound is necessary at that point. If I am in the grocery store and hear a child screaming, it is typically dismissed as somebody's bratty little kid throwing a fit because they didn't get their way.

However, if a child screams "STRANGER!" everyone in earshot will be turning their attention to that child. The same goes for women in a public setting. If you are being threatened, don't hesitate to lower your tone and raise your voice. Just saying "NO!" can sometimes be enough to stop a would-be attacker.

Emergency phrases such as "FIRE!", "911!", "LEAVE ME ALONE!" can get the attention of those around you as well as make an attacker think twice. That, along with a defensive posturing make for strong language, both body and verbal.

Another thing to consider is that the word "NO" is a complete sentence. It does not require explanation or justification. If you are in a relationship with someone and you have been intimate with them before, but, this time you decide that you do not wish to be so, then No is the response.

If someone does NOT take *No* for an answer, then they have just told you that they do not respect you. Simple as that. No means no. A major red flag should go up in your head if someone does not or will not take no for an answer.

Whether it is someone you just met who wants to buy you a drink, or someone you work with that keeps asking you out- if they are not respectful or your boundaries, they are trouble. Make your boundaries crystal clear, with a straight-forward approach so there is no room for doubt. Everyone interprets things differently.

If you encounter someone who is socially awkward, or aggressive or just plain clueless, then, the polite approach probably won't work. Be blunt. Surprisingly enough, some people are not offended by that approach at all; in fact, it's what they understand.

I had a teenage student once that was really a nice guy at heart, but socially awkward. A highly intelligent soul, he was very analytical and a left brained thinker. But, he did love the ladies, and looked forward to chatting with them after class. To him, he was just interested in them and wanted to get to know them. To the girls, he was a wolf cornering his prey! After I observed him sitting with a young lady who looked like she was cornered, I called him over and she made her escape.
I had a semi-lengthy conversation with this young man about this particular behavior and he was, quite frankly, clueless.

I took a passive approach initially, but quickly realized that was not going to cut it with him. So, I told him bluntly to leave the girls alone, to not pursue them after class and not ask them for their phone numbers or anything else. It worked. He understood this approach and was not offended at all.

Even if he had been, it was necessary to change his behavior since it was making the female students uncomfortable. Eventually, he matured and formed healthy relationships with women and is to this day a respectable and polite man.

Self-defense is not just about being physically attacked. It is about protecting yourself from emotional harm, too. When someone makes you uncomfortable, it is your perfect right to speak up. It is your right to say something about their behavior that is making you uncomfortable, or to get up and walk away. No explanation necessary.

Many times, men will try your defenses with little comments or even physical approaches to "test the waters." If you don't say no right away, then in their mind, you said yes. The next time it goes further- little by little - until they have gotten what they wanted from you. Whether it is control, dominance- or something more.

In an abusive relationship, most times it didn't start out with abusive behavior. The prince of darkness started out as prince charming. The little things that he did that annoyed you were often overlooked or dismissed because he was so charming and attentive in every other way.

Likely your definition of being the bigger person and overlooking his quirks was taken as a sign of weakness by him and he zeroed in on it.

Setting boundaries with people is a healthy thing. It is necessary for children to develop in a positive environment, it is necessary for a relationship to survive in a healthy way and it is important in a healthy work environment, too. You teach people how to treat you. Your actions- or inactions teach people just how far they can go with you in any given situation.

There are always going to be people in this world who are more than willing to take advantage of you, if you let them. It is up to you to set and keep healthy boundaries. No guilt, no shame, no fear. No justification necessary. It is your perfect right.

Saying yes when you really want to say no is being a victim.

Saying no when you want to say no is refusing to be a victim any longer. We have learned behaviors throughout our lives and fallen into patterns that sometimes we are not even aware of.

Changing a habit, any habit, takes time and practice. If you are uncomfortable enough saying no that you say yes instead, then it's time to re-evaluate your situation. Make a plan as to how you are going to change that unhealthy habit. Start small and build.

Practice with someone you trust. Why would you expect more from yourself than you would expect from others? Why would you give others more credit than you give yourself? Give yourself permission to say no.

MOST ATTACKS HAPPEN IN TRANSIT

At my training center, I spoke with a mother of one of my former students who had been attacked on her way to work. After she parked in the company parking lot, she was walking towards her building when a car pulled up, a man jumped out from the passenger side and punched her, knocking her down and taking her purse.

We had been talking about carrying mace, which she did. I asked her where it was and she told me it was on her keychain, in the cute little pink leather case. Meaning-- it was not accessible. She wasn't ready to use it. Just like any weapon, it is useless if you can't get to it.

Most attacks happen in transit, such as walking from your car to your house, from the shopping center to your car, etc. You have to have whatever you are depending on as a weapon ready to use. If your mace is locked in a case with the safety on, or in the bottom of your purse, it is useless.

An attack happens in a matter of seconds. There are a wide variety of mace and pepper spray products on the market today. The "triple threat" version contains mace, pepper spray and a dye. The dye is the same type banks use to explode in the money bag if they are robbed. So, if you spray the bad guy with this version, he will burn, itch and be marked for easy identification.

Many people have heard that you should carry your keys in your hand by sticking the longest keys between your fingers. Personally, I think exposing one large key between the fingers is plenty. You can hit with a closed fist and jab the key into your attacker that way without the opportunity to squeeze your fingers together and hurt yourself if multiple keys are exposed.

Another really good device to add to your keychain is a kubotan. A kubotan is basically a stick that you can hold firmly and one end holds your keys, which are great for striking across an attackers face/eyes and the other end is a solid point that can be used to strike with as well.
It is much more stable than a key between the fingers, is a harder surface to hit with and is very effective, if used properly. They can be made of wood, but some are made of aluminum steel and some even have prongs that extend so it can be carried for use on either end or with the prongs, which are protruding between the fingers but can't be squeezed together like keys might be.

Like any weapon, they cannot be carried into a courthouse, airport, or other federal properties among other places.

ARMS, LEGS AND VOICE

There was a story several years back about a little girl who was attacked while walking home from her aunt's house which was just around the corner from hers. As her attacker picked her up, she remembered what her father had taught her: If someone grabs you, just wiggle and scream. So, when her attacker grabbed her and picked her up, she started wiggling and screaming for all she was worth. It worked.

The 18 year old male that had grabbed her, dropped her and she took off running. She made it home, the police were called and the assailant was captured. There is a lot to be said for wiggling and screaming.

There was another case of an elderly woman who woke up one evening to find a man on top of her. She knew that he could overpower her, so the only thing she felt she could do was "grab and twist". She grabbed his groin, held on tight and twisted as hard as she could. Her attacker, who was in great pain, punched her several times, but she didn't let go. She held on as they struggled off the bed, down the hall and towards the front door.

He passed out several times in the process, begged for her to let go, call the police-- anything to get relief from the excruciating pain he felt, but, she didn't let up. When he finally got the front door unlocked, she let go and he ran into the night…. leaving behind his wallet.

The police had no problem catching up with him. One simple technique saved this woman's life. There's something to be said for the "grab and twist" technique.

USE WHAT YOU HAVE AND KNOW
YOU WILL USE

This is a big one. Anything around you can be used as a weapon. If you can pick it up, knock it over, hide behind it, it can be a weapon. During a seminar, a woman gave testimony as to an incident that had happened to her in her home. Someone banged on the door and she got scared, looked around for a weapon and the only thing within her reach was a yardstick in the umbrella stand by the door.

She grabbed the yardstick, feeling foolish and opened the door. It turned out to be a harmless encounter, but had it been something more, her question was, "What was I going to do with a yardstick?" So, I showed her.

After we discussed the fact that the doorbell and the phone are conveniences and do not require that you answer them... I described how the ends of the stick are a much harder surface to hit with, and the vital points that can be used to disable an attacker.

Then, like using the blade of a sword, I demonstrated the stability of the yardstick by breaking a board with it. She was shocked. But, if you know where to hit, you can use anything as either a weapon or a distraction.

We then discussed about advanced planning and I recommended that she go through her house and just see what could possibly be used as a weapon, should the need arise. That way, anywhere she was in her house, she had an idea of what was available to her and how to use it.

Then, we discussed how pepper spray canisters can be velcroed behind doors, in the kitchen, the shower and anywhere she felt she could have quick access without it being in an obvious place throughout her house and vehicle.

Many fitness buffs have taken to walking for their health, which is a great idea. But, a few simple precautions should be taken while exercising outdoors. First, dress appropriately. Not only for the weather, but for the spectators, too. You have every right to dress however you feel is best for you, but, know that the more revealing the attire, the more attention it will garnish. It's just the way it is.

So, if you are trying to avoid unwanted attention, dress accordingly. Sweat pants may be too hot for the middle of the summer, but loose shorts that hide the essentials are better than short shorts that are tight and attention grabbing. A sports bra may be cooler and more comfortable for that summer jog, but it may not be the best idea.

A cotton t-shirt can wick away the moisture and will draw less attention. That being said, it is important to remember that attackers are many times more enticed by situation, and not the physical appeal of the victim. Whether you weigh 100 pounds or 300 pounds may not be the deciding factor as to whether an attacker picks you as his next victim, but your vulnerability may be.

If you are a target that is too good to pass up in the mind of an attacker (meaning- you were distracted, not aware and didn't look like you would put up much of a fight, if any) then you are prime target material.

On the other hand, if you are alert, aware and ready, your chances of being attacked go down significantly. In our program, we teach each member how to use a short stick, sometimes called an escrima stick. It is a lightweight, hardwood stick that is easy to carry. It is long enough to be an extension of your body, but short enough that it is hard to take away from the owner.

Our GET REAL sticks come in a bright, safety yellow color which can be seen not only by traffic, but would be attackers. Just being ready is a deterrent.

San Antonio is home to several military bases. Some years back, when wireless headphones were a big deal, two female cadets went for a jog, one wearing headphones. About a mile into the run, the cadet without the headset decided to turn back and the other jogger kept going.

The young lady wearing the headset never made it back to the barracks. As she ran with her headphones, a truck pulled up beside her and two men jumped out, kidnapped her, raped her and killed her, leaving her body in a field just a short distance from the road.

Her headphones not only made her less aware of what was going on around her, they also made her *look* less aware. It was a costly and tragic mistake.
If you are going to be exercising outdoors, be aware of what is going on around you and let others see that you are aware of them.

If you are facing traffic, you can see what is coming and have a better chance to get out of the way, should you have to. If traffic is at your back, you can be seen *by* them, but you can't see them.

Your reaction time is greatly reduced. Always face traffic if you are walking or jogging. Bicycle laws differ from state to state, but usually they have to adhere to the same traffic laws as motored vehicles. Be sure and check your local laws if you are a bike rider. Either way- be prepared.

FINAL THOUGHTS ON THIS SECTION

The next section of this book will deal with the physical aspects of defending oneself. Please keep in mind that your mental state has much to do with your physical state. If you are going to defend yourself physically, be prepared to "give it all you've got."

My hope is that you can take away from this book the mental and emotional tools you can develop to keep you from ever having to defend your life with your physical skills.

But, if the time does come that you have no choice but to physically defend yourself, then the tools in this next section are there for you, too.

Earlier in this book, I quoted the line, "It's not the size of the dog in the fight, it's the size of the fight in the dog" that matters. It's true. Your attitude affects your physical performance.

In the case of using deadly force, such as a firearm, the theory is that if you are going to shoot, then shoot to kill. If someone is attacking you with deadly force, pick the largest mass- the midsection- and empty the clip. It's too hard to pick a non-lethal target, say, the left kneecap, when someone is running at you or beating on you or whatever.

The same goes for using your body as a weapon: EMPTY THE CLIP! Do not hit once and stop, expecting it to work like it does in the movies... it won't. It will hurt you to hit a solid object- especially if you've never really hit anything with such force.

If your life depended on it, give it everything you've got and don't stop until you are able to get away to safety. The ideal situation is to get into some kind of self- defense based course where you can build your strength, knowledge and stamina along with your technical skills.

If you are going to carry a hand gun, or you have guns in your home, then consider taking a course. There are certification courses available as well as strictly skills development courses. The more you know, the more confident you are.

What we're going to go through in this next section will give you a solid foundation on which to build your physical arsenal.

9 ESCAPES

RELEASES

There are three basic levels of physical self- defense.

1-Escape
2- Control
3- Destroy

Let's talk about #1- Escape.

If escaping is an option, it is always your best option. If someone grabs you, it is because they thought they could take you.   Men are biologically bigger and stronger than women, so fighting strength against strength is a losing battle for most.   So, let's think from a different angle.

If someone reaches out their arm and grabs you, their strength comes from a straight wrist and the strength of their fingers. The weakest part of the grip is the thumb.

 Think of it this way. If you were to hang on the monkey bars, you could hang with just your fingers, but, you couldn't hang with just your thumbs. So, the thumb is the target for a release. Whether you pull away from your attacker, or you pull back their thumb and release yourself, your focus is the thumb.

Now, when you are first learning any technique, developing good technique is the key, not speed or strength. Try each technique in slow motion and without resistance until you feel more comfortable. Of course, if someone grabs you, they will be using full resistance.

But, for practice purposes, little or no resistance is the way to learn the techniques, gain some confidence and perfect the moves. The more resistance there is, the more force is required to escape. Meaning, the opportunity for injury to either the attacker or the victim or both is greater with greater resistance.

Until you feel more confident with any technique, work on it slowly, with little or no resistance.

When someone throws a punch, or a kick, or reaches out to grab another person, it is typically in a semi-linear movement. One way to counter the impact of a linear attack is with circular movements.

For instance, if someone grabs your arm, they have reached out and are either pushing or pulling your arm. If you take your wrists and make small circles, you will have more ability to release yourself from their grip than if you tried to swing your whole arm away.

Once you make a circle, either clockwise or counterclockwise, you will eventually get to the point where it is the thumb of the attacker that is what they are trying to hang on to you with. Fingertips are not very strong, especially if the wrist is bent.

For example, have you ever lifted something like a big pickle jar? As you pick it up off the counter you have a straight wrist with full grip. As you lift the jar to put it into the cabinet, you reach a point where the wrist bends and suddenly you don't have the strength you had below eye level.

It is just fingertips hanging on and the other hand instinctively comes to the rescue to grab the bottom of the jar so it doesn't fall. That point where the wrist bent is where the strength left. This is the point where martial artists use to escape grips.

Making small circles, snake your fingertips around the attackers arm until you free yourself. The good thing is, you can't go the wrong way-either way you go, you will eventually get to the point where the thumb is the main resistance and you can get free.

Now, not everything works every time and not everything works on everybody. If Plan A doesn't work, go immediately to Plan B. Go through the alphabet if you have to, but just don't quit until you are free.

The basic circle is effective in many situations. If someone chokes you, you have just a few seconds before you pass out if they are squeezing you. In Judo, it takes less than 5 seconds to choke an opponent unconscious. If someone gets their hands on your neck, you have to react and you have to react fast.

A choke is a more life threatening attack and a simple escape may not do the trick. Although circular motions can still be employed, they may need to be preceded or followed with some effective strikes, which we will discuss a little later on.

For now, let's look at some circular movements to escape a choke. The only good thing about someone having their hands on your neck is you know that they aren't going to punch you while they are grabbing you. The bad part is, they are choking you. Now, if someone grabs you, again, they think they are in control. They have used the element of surprise and are feeling dominant. If you don't react at all, you will likely pass out in a matter of seconds.

If you push into the attack, you make that passing out happen even faster since you are applying even more pressure on your throat. Instinctively, you want to get away from the attack, so you pull back. Remember, the strength of the grip is the four fingers, and, in a choke, you have 8 of them around your neck. Pulling back is not the best option in and of itself.

But, if as you pull back, you swing one arm over the top of both of his arms and turn your body to the side, you will be able to push his grip down and away from your neck, releasing the grip.

If you grab one arm, step back with the same foot and swing the opposite arm over the top of his arms, you will not only release his grip, but you will pull him forward, off-balancing him and you can clamp your swinging arm down on his two arms as they slide off your neck, resulting in a controlling situation.

Your body is turned to the side and you have just trapped his arms. The motion of your twisting hips has not only pulled you away from his grip, it has pulled him off balance. As his momentum is still traveling forward, immediately twist your hips back into him, bringing your elbow into his face at the same time.

If you are still hanging on with the first hand that you grabbed him with, you can pull with that hand as you push with your other elbow and get even more power into your strike. Like any other technique, it takes practice to get the hang of it, but, once you do, it is a very effective defense. This whole scenario takes less than a second or two to execute full force.

If someone gets their hands around your neck, you have to react quickly, as we talked about before. 360 degrees around the neck is a vulnerable spot to get choked or hit. If you are being choked, try to get your chin down to your chest to protect your windpipe.

If you can get your head underneath one arm, you can turn out to that side and get out of the grip. It's the same concept as an alligator rolling to disable its prey.

Another concept I want you to embrace is the "it's mine, I'm keeping it" concept of self-defense. Whether they consciously think about it or not, an attacker is expecting you to put up some kind of a fight.

They are expecting you to be surprised by their attack and they are expecting to win. With that being said, what they are not expecting is someone to overpower them.

They didn't pick on someone they thought would kick their butt- they picked on someone because they thought the odds were in their favor for winning that confrontation.

In the "it's mine, I'm keeping it" concept of self- defense, when someone reaches out and grabs you, whatever they extended to you becomes "yours."

For instance, if someone grabs my hair, my instinct might be to get them off of me as quickly as possible. But, the drawback with that approach is I will lose whatever hair is in the attackers hand(s) when I do.

So, if I pull their hand INTO my head and hang on to their hand with my hands, then I am preventing them from pulling out my hair while I am becoming the attacker and taking control of the situation. I can follow up several different ways.

First, if I want to strike, I have my legs free. But, if I want to immobilize my attacker, I can turn the arm I am taking possession of into a locked position, called an arm bar. Chances are, just about anywhere someone grabs you, they can apply an arm bar.

Your body has joints such as wrists, elbows, shoulders, etc. that can be locked to immobilize an attacker.
If you watch mixed martial arts, (MMA) at all, you will see lots of arm locks being applied. It is an effective way to stop an opponent.

Take your elbow, for example. It is meant to bend in two directions. Once you get to the full extension of your arm, your elbow is locked. If it goes any further, it will either hyper extend or dislocate, depending on the amount of force applied. If you have ever thrown a punch, you might have hyper-extended your own elbow.

It only takes about four pounds of pressure to dislocate an elbow, so it is a prime spot for joint locks. If someone grabs you, chances are, you can take that arm and turn it into an arm bar. It is not a complicated move, but it does take practice.   There are both straight arm bars and bent arm bars, depending on whether the elbow is locked (straight) or bent.

Let's take another grab. Let's say an attacker grabs your lapel. First, you take your hands and put them around your attacker's wrist. Pull him into your chest and push your chest into his hand. While doing this, turn your body towards the outside of your opponent for a straight arm bar.

As you move your body around in a circular motion, bring your elbow over his elbow. The closer you are, the more control you will have. To determine which side of your opponent you should move towards, remember that the locking side of the elbow is on the pinky side of their hand. That is, the elbow bends toward the thumb, so putting pressure on the side where the pinky is will result in the elbow locking.

If I grab my opponent's wrist with both hands, pulling their hand into my chest while stepping back and turning my hip towards the outside of the elbow, I can pull my opponent off balance.

If I bring my outside elbow over his elbow and apply pressure downward and keep my back straight at the same time, I will push my opponent's head downward. At this point, his shoulder is lower than his hand, his balance is off and his arm is locked.

I can either push him off and start running at this point, or I can follow through until he is on the ground. If I choose to stick around and fight, I need to be kicking, kneeing and striking him and breaking that elbow I was holding on to.

In a classroom situation, we practice arm locks and joint locks with little or no resistance and very little speed so that we can avoid injuries and keep practicing, perfecting the techniques. In a self- defense situation, these same techniques can be applied full speed, not only bringing down an opponent, but breaking bones in the process.

STRIKES

First, let's talk about what we have on us or around us that can be used as a weapon to strike an opponent. Basically, if you can pick it up, it can be used as a weapon! If you are sitting at a desk, say in an office, look around you.

What do you see that could be used to strike someone with? A pen, pencil, stapler, coaster, a phone, calculator, paper clips, marker or book? These are things on my desk right now that could be used in some way to defend myself. Even if it is only used as a distraction, it is still a valuable weapon should the need arise.

Let's say we are out and the only weapons we have are ourselves. Fine. Our bodies are an arsenal of weapons if we know where and how to use them. Let's start at the top: our head. The skull is the thickest bone in our bodies, to protect our brains. This can be used quite effectively as a weapon.
Let's say someone attacks you from behind, say, a bear hug style attack.

The back of the head can be used to strike the attackers nose, face, or side of the head quite effectively. The shoulder can be used in close range to strike with also.

The chin is a prime target for a shoulder thrust. Teeth clashing together at a high rate of speed can be quite painful for an unsuspecting opponent.
The arms are the most natural of weapons, since we use them for most everything we do every day.

Elbows, forearms and hands can be used as weapons quite effectively with a little training.
Knees, legs and feet can also be conditioned to strike with bone breaking, opponent stopping force.

We will be demonstrating several techniques in the chapter on striking that are designed for maximum efficiency, minimum effort.

With that being said, let's talk a bit about actually hitting a target, whether it be in practice or in a crisis situation. We are by nature, very visual creatures and have all witnessed scenarios of physical confrontations, whether it was in movies or on TV or otherwise.

Visualizing is an important component for successful training in martial arts, or any sport, but, it doesn't compare to the actual feeling of getting hit or hitting something or someone for real.

The saying goes, "everyone has a plan until they get punched in the face". The sudden shock of actually getting hit, along with the physical pain it instantly inflicts, is often so overwhelming that people freeze or crumble.

One of the benefits of taking a self- defense class or seminar is that you actually get to hit something! Even hitting a practice target that is covered in foam is enough to trigger your body to have a more automatic response when pain is involved. We don't want our bodies to freeze in the event an actual attack occurs. There is no doubt that in the event of an actual attack, you are going to get hurt. The difference is, how bad?

I would much rather my students get bumped and bruised in practice than get seriously injured or killed in a real attack. By using their knees to hit one of our "bad guys" dressed in full body armor, our students will probably leave with fabric burns and/or bruises where they made contact.

They may skin their elbows or have some other minor aches by the time they leave, but the difference is distinct-- no one is INJURED. And, they all got a chance to actually feel what it took to stop someone in an attack, since our instructors will only cease their attacks when they feel the strikes were effective enough to stop them if they weren't wearing protective gear.

Another aspect of hands-on training that most every participant comments on after the fact, is that they knew they were in a safe environment while training, they knew the attacker was going to use some level of control and they knew this was a mock situation, yet it was still shocking to them when they got grabbed. And although they were surprised that they were surprised they didn't stop!

They kicked and screamed and struck their attacker and yelled and made every effort to get free until they were. They used their whole bodies as weapons to get away as soon as possible.

Although it can be a scary situation, it is so empowering for each participant to actually see, in real time, that they have the ability to stop an attacker. Although everyone is in a different state of physical fitness or physical readiness, everyone has the ability to defend themselves in some way.

It's great that you are reading this book. I'm grateful to have the opportunity to give you some things to think about, to educate you and to motivate you. But, going out and actually participating in a self-defense class brings you up to a whole new level of abilities, empowerment and confidence.

After reading this book, I hope you will reach out to your community and seek out a class. Sometimes they are offered at facilities like martial arts or fitness centers, sometimes they are on college campuses or school campuses associated with continuing education programs. Community centers sometimes have them available, too. Look around. If you can't find anything nearby, then check our website, or send me an email and we will help you find something or set something up.

The importance of having some physical practice in the event that an attack reaches the final stage- which is the physical attack- is imperative. It can increase your chances of survival significantly.
But, remember, the awareness aspect of self- defense is there to keep you from reaching the final stage of an attack. But, for whatever reason, should you find yourself in the final stage, the physical stage, of an attack, it is time to fight for your life. Literally.

PRESSURE POINTS

Pressure points are nerve endings. Like hitting your funny bone- (which is never funny, by the way!) nerve endings are our sensors. If you have ever been fortunate enough to have a good massage, then you have had your nerves gently manipulated for healing and relaxation purposes.

If you have had acupuncture, the nerves have been stimulated by tiny needles to facilitate healing. But, if significant blunt force is applied to those same nerve endings, or pressure points, then a very different result occurs. Extreme overstimulation will cause temporary or permanent damage, depending on the force applied.

For example, if you turned on every electrical appliance in your house on at the same time, you would likely cause a black out- the fuses blow due to system overload.

If you have ever watched a boxing match, for instance, and you see a fighter get punched in the head and his knees buckle, that is the same type of system overload. Everything in our bodies are connected electrically.

If you get hit in the head with enough force, you can become unconscious before your legs give out and you fall to the ground. If the blow is severe enough, then permanent damage or even death can occur.

In self- defense, pressure points are used to either temporarily or permanently disable an attacker. They can be used to release a grip, they can be used to control the attacker, or they can be used to disable them, depending on the amount of force used, as well as the location of the hit.

Pressure points are also a favorable weapon for self- defense because they don't require a great deal of strength to be used effectively. It's not always how hard you hit someone that matters, it's where you hit them that counts.

Imagine going to the beach and seeing a big, burly guy walking along the sand. Now, imagine a single grain of sand in his eye. Chances are, that tiny grain of sand is going to consume all of his attention until it is OUT of his eye! The eyes are such sensitive areas they do not require much force to damage.

Imagine taking one finger or your thumb and jabbing it into an attacker's eye. It would not require great strength to execute this self-defense move, but it would yield enormous results.

PRIME TARGET AREAS

The closer you go towards the center line of your body, the more lethal the blow. The further away from the center line, the less lethal the blow. For example, if you took a baseball bat and struck it over my arm, you would break my arm, but, I'm not going to die from the blow. However, the same amount of force with the same baseball bat over my head just might result in death. Same force, different spot, totally different result.

So, if you are going to strike someone in a life and death situation, make it count. Don't waste time and energy hitting someone ineffectively. It is not the size of what you strike with or even the force with which you strike, but where you strike that counts most.

Even a big opponent can be stopped with a grain of sand in their eye. Your thumbs are bigger than a grain of sand, but they will stop someone pretty fast!

Our sight is one of our senses that we depend on the most. We could all function pretty "normally" (whatever normal means) without our sense of smell, or even our hearing, but, take away our sight and the game is changed.

So, striking to and about the eyes is an effective move. If you can get your hands to their head, stick your thumbs in their eyes. I know this sounds gross, but the eyes are a ball rolling around in a socket, basically.

If you apply pressure from the inside to the outside, you can make someone's eye(s) pop out. I guarantee you, if you pop out someone's eyes, they are no longer concerned with pursuing you!

Along that center line of your head lies your nose. Have you ever gotten hit in the nose? Wow, it hurts. It makes your eyes water, and it can temporarily immobilize an attacker. It doesn't take a lot of force to break someone's nose.

Actually, my daughter broke mine with the back of her head when she was 18 months old! She pulled away from who was grabbing for her and, although I was lying in bed, almost asleep, her head came across my nose from the side and broke it. It didn't take a lot, but it certainly made for a rude awakening!

Have you ever slapped someone? If you use the end of your hand, your fingers will leave a big red mark on their face and chances are they are going to be really mad after that slap. That's about the extent of the damage.

 But, if you use the same amount of force and strike a few inches further down your hand with the palm of your hand, that force can potentially break their jaw or their nose!

Same movement, same force- different results.   If you use the same motion as a volleyball player would use to spike a ball, striking the nose in a downward angle with the base of the palm of the hand, it will break the nose.

That same strike can be effective to the side of the temple, the ears and the base of the jaw right under the ears.

Moving down the center line of the body is the throat area. There are vulnerable spots all the way around the neck, so let's start in the front. The windpipe is made of cartilage, and is shaped something like the tube on a vacuum cleaner. If you strike the windpipe, it doesn't take much force before the throat seizes and the person will be gasping for air.

You can strike with the fist, but you have to have a strong wrist to avoid self- injury. If you are close enough, hit them with the blade of your forearm between the wrist and elbow- it's much stronger. Or, just grab their throat and try and touch your fingers together behind the windpipe.
One of the strongest hand techniques for women to strike with is the hammer fist. Close your fist and use the padded part on the outside

between your pinky finger and your wrist, just like you would if you were pounding on your desk.

This hammer can be used to strike downward, like striking the nose and/or collarbone. It can be used to strike the groin, especially if someone is grabbing you from behind. Although the elbow is very strong, the hammer fist gains you more reach and leverage when striking the groin from behind.

If you are striking someone who is standing to your side, the hammer fist is a strong weapon. If you are closer than you thought, the forearm is there and is a great tool.

Think of your arm like a sword. It's long and thin and the sharp part along the edge is the blade. The stronger blade is along the outside of your arm, on the pinky side. That is the forearm and it is a great weapon. It is what martial artists use to block kicks and punches with quite effectively and it can also be used to strike targets for self-defense purposes quite well.

Moving down from the throat, along the center line of the body is the sternum, or chest area. Where your ribs meet in the front, there is the sternum bone, a small bone that protrudes downward about an inch or so. If struck with the palm of the hand, or the point of the elbow, this little bone could break and potentially puncture a lung, causing a great deal of pain and damage or even death.

Moving down the center line of the body we reach the all-sensitive groin area. Granted, men and boys learn early on in life that this is an extremely sensitive area if they get hit.

Thus, they develop quite extraordinarily fast reflexes with either the "knee up and leg across the groin" move or the "catcher's mitt" hand approach to protecting their family jewels.

None the less, a swift knee, hammer fist, kick or "grab and twist" technique can be most effective in dropping an attacker when applied to the groin.

Moving down the inside of the legs, the inner thighs (like the inner arms) are highly sensitive areas for a pinch, while the knees are prime targets for kicks.

The shins, if raked down with the side of a shoe or kicked with the bottom of the foot, can be extremely painful targets of attack.

The tops of the feet can be stomped on with the heel of a shoe, which can actually break the small bones on the top of the foot.

EMPTY THE CLIP!

Just like shooting an automatic weapon, your strikes should be forceful, concentrated and continuous. Palm heels to the nose can be thrown 4-6 times within a one second time frame.

Kicking, punching, screaming-- let it all out and go all out and do not stop until you are able to get away to safety. As soon as you can drop an opponent or create some space, try and escape. Until then, empty the clip!

10 BECOME A BLACK BELT IN AWARENESS

BECOME A BLACK BELT IN AWARENESS

Unless you are wearing your karate uniform and black belt, no one knows you are a skilled fighter while you are pushing a grocery cart down the produce aisle. And, it would look a little strange if you did.

However, you can become a black belt in awareness without the degree. Paying conscious attention to what is going on around you will increase your awareness skills. Taking the next step and acting on them will enhance your awareness skills even more.

There is a private school nearby that has alert and responsible teachers, administrators and staff all around. The local police patrol the area frequently and a disaster plan is in effect and practiced regularly.

By all accounts, this group of caretakers is doing a good job and being aware. But, sometimes our awareness needs to be amplified and exercised. An officer decided to patrol the area one day and run his own experiment. He pulled up in an unmarked car which had dark tinted windows.

He slowly approached the area and stopped, then moved up a bit and stopped again. Several teachers made their body language clear that they saw the suspicious driver and were aware of his presence. Their fight or flight instincts looked to be intact. However, that's as far as it went. They didn't approach the vehicle- wisely. But, they didn't alert the authorities either. Each teacher is equipped with a cell phone and a direct line to the local police should something occur.

That one extra step is a major component to ensuring safety. Not dismissing their concern, or invalidating their intuition, but taking that next step. In a worst case scenario, it could mean stopping a violent attack on the school. In the best case scenario, it turns out to be nothing. Either way, it is a win/win situation.

The good news in this story is that it was an officer with good intent who was training the teachers to react when they felt a possible threat.

Like running a fire drill, it is an exercise in safety. We learn from practice what works and what doesn't, and we modify as needed.

HIGHER AWARENESS LESSENS ANXIETY

Anxiety is a fear of the unknown. When you are not aware of your surroundings, you are also less capable of responding in a competent manner.

When you pay attention to the details of what's going on around you, you are less likely to be taken by total surprise and less likely to panic in a crisis. If you are mentally prepared, you are
able to react more rapidly should the situation turn into a fight or flight scenario. For instance, I've been a competent driver for many years now.

At the age of 16, when I got my license, I was much more nervous about getting on the highway or merging with traffic than I am today. It's experience that keeps me calm. The traffic hasn't changed but my skills have.

Then, several years ago, I took a motorcycle safety course when I bought my first bike. After completing that course, I became an even better driver because riding a bike required I be more aware. There are no seat belts or air bags on a motorcycle. Your level of awareness instantly goes up when you get on a bike.

The 3-second rule of looking ahead goes to 11-seconds. You start looking at things with fresh eyes.
Personal safety is like riding a bike. You should definitely enjoy the ride, but dress for the crash. Be aware, be prepared, but don't let the fear stop you from getting out and experiencing what life has to offer.

The more you practice being aware, the calmer you become. The more confident you become that you can handle situations that might arise, because you've thought about what to do in case of an emergency and you have formulated some kind of a plan. Even if it's a rough outline, it's still better than no plan at all.

IT'S NOT HOW MUCH YOU KNOW, BUT HOW WELL YOU KNOW IT

You don't have to be a world champion or an MMA fighter to defend yourself. Knowing just a few key skills and tactics can save your life.

Even though you can always increase your arsenal- and I encourage you to do that- it's not how many techniques you know that can make the difference in your safety.

It's the ability to execute one or two effective techniques with precision that are life savers. The more you know, the more confident you can become. But, when it comes down to it, the most basic things work the best.

ACT ON YOUR INSTINCTS

That inner voice, your internal body guard, is there to protect you. Practice listening. The more you trust your instincts, the more balanced your life will be. Take baby steps at first, but act on what your inner voice is telling you is right for you. With practice, this voice will get louder and stronger, and so will you. Acting on your instincts can be the single most effective tool in your personal safety arsenal.

BE ASSERTIVE

If you are not naturally assertive, it's not too late to start. "To thine own self be true." Know what you want. Big or small, what you want does matter. Give yourself the respect you give to others. Give yourself the respect you want others to give you. Do not tolerate disrespectful behavior. Tell the truth. Whether it's "That hurts my feelings", or "I don't like that", or "I'm not going to do that." "No." No means no. There is no need for explanation. Speak up. You will feel better and better about yourself the more you do.

FAKE IT TILL YOU MAKE IT

Others take at face value what you present more times than not. If you present yourself as assertive, confident and relaxed, that's typically what others will assume you are. If you present yourself as weak, timid and shy, that's what others will assume you to be. It reflects in your body language as well as your speech and actions. Whatever energy you project is what the world will consume.

If you aren't happy with the way the world treats you, then decide to project a different energy. First, see yourself as a strong, confident, assertive woman. Visualize it; see yourself in great detail going through your day as a vibrant, successful, knowledgeable, able-bodied woman. If you want to be one, you have to *act* like one, *train* like one and eventually   you   will   *BE*   one.

ABOUT THE AUTHOR

Rhonda Payne is a full time martial arts instructor at the House of Payne, Inc. in Converse, TX. She conducts seminars for Get REAL and can be contacted at info@getrealsafety.com.

CPSIA information can be obtained at www.ICGtesting.com
Printed in the USA
LVOW01s2027191014

409476LV00018BB/1007/P